# EXERCISE MEDICINE FOR THE FRAILTY SYNDROME

Frailty is a clinical syndrome caused by multiple chronic conditions that makes it difficult to maintain homeostasis. In part, it is the result of the body's inability to regulate normal inflammatory responses that lead to muscle loss, decrease in strength, and independence. Regular exercise helps to optimize physiological performance. It is a profound influence, especially in the presence of physical inactivity, where the lack of exercise leads to poor health and decreased longevity. Unfortunately, a high percentage of Americans fail to engage in daily exercise with the older population becoming increasingly frail, which is a syndrome characterized by declines in musculoskeletal and physiologic reserve and function. It has been documented that exercise is medicine and can be better than the effects induced by drugs. Exercise physiologists are healthcare professionals. They are key professionals in developing and applying an exercise medicine prescription for frail adults.

*Exercise Medicine for the Frailty Syndrome* speaks to the benefits of exercise medicine as the best therapy to prevent or reverse the age-related muscle loss and functional deficits that are predictive of an increase in falls, hospitalization, institutionalization, and mortality. This book is a proactive step to help increase the functional independence of older frail adults. It highlights Board Certification by the American Society of Exercise Physiologists as the professional qualification to improve society's understanding of the biological treatment and complexity of the frailty syndrome and is key reading for Exercise Physiologists.

**Tommy Boone**, PhD, MPH, MAM, MBA, FASEP, EPC, is a founding member and first President of the American Society of Exercise Physiologists (ASEP).

# EXERCISE MEDICINE FOR THE FRAILTY SYNDROME

*Tommy Boone*

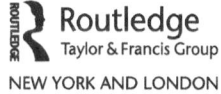

Routledge
Taylor & Francis Group

NEW YORK AND LONDON

Cover image: Shutterstock

First published 2023
by Routledge
605 Third Avenue, New York, NY 10158

and by Routledge
4 Park Square, Milton Park, Abingdon, Oxon, OX14 4RN

*Routledge is an imprint of the Taylor & Francis Group, an informa business*

*Library of Congress Cataloging-in-Publication Data*
A catalog record for this book has been requested

ISBN: 978-0-367-63603-6 (hbk)
ISBN: 978-0-367-63600-5 (pbk)
ISBN: 978-1-003-11992-0 (ebk)

DOI: 10.4324/9781003119920

Typeset in Bembo
by Apex CoVantage, LLC

# CONTENTS

# BOXES

# FOREWORD

While there is little to no consensus on the definition of frailty, Dr. Boone has addressed the phenotype of frailty and identified the clinical concerns of older adults. He has also presented a sound physiological argument for a successful prevention and/or treatment for frailty, which is exercise medicine. Like many things exercise physiologists deal with in health care, developing and applying an exercise medicine prescription to frail adults is on one hand a straightforward physiological assessment and application and on the other hand a multifactorial process given that frailty implies vulnerability.

*Exercise Medicine for the Frailty Syndrome* presents an important analysis of the combination of specific symptoms and, in particular, sarcopenia that is recognized as a major component of frailty. The content speaks to the benefits of exercise medicine as the best therapy to prevent and reverse the age-related muscle loss and functional deficits that are predictive of an increase in falls, hospitalization, institutionalization, and mortality.

While the students of exercise physiology are presently being taught the beneficial effects of exercise, especially in terms of atherosclerosis, diabetes, hypertension, and depression, Dr. Boone's emphasis on exercise medicine as the prescriptive method for preventing and treating (i.e., possibly reversing) frailty is a professional proactive step to increase functional independence of older adults.

Dr. Boone identifies numerous studies in support of his views regarding increased muscular mobility, improved gait and bone mineral density, enhanced performance of daily activities, and fewer falls and hospitalizations. Also, he highlights the ASEP Board-Certified Exercise Physiologists as important healthcare professionals in the fight to improve the health and well-being of the elderly frail adults via the exercise medicine prescription.

Dr. Frank B. Wyatt, EPC, FASEP
Department of Athletic Training & Exercise Physiology
Midwestern State University
Wichita Falls, TX

# PREFACE

Frailty is a clinical syndrome caused by multiple chronic conditions that makes it difficult to maintain homeostasis. In part, it is the result of the body's inability to regulate normal inflammatory responses that lead to muscle loss, decrease in strength, and independence. Frailty can severely influence quality of life, as well as increase the burden placed on the family and society. The syndrome driven by a sedentary lifestyle has increasingly attracted attention of researchers, healthcare community, and the exercise physiology profession. Fortunately, exercise physiologists are in position to prescribe the aerobic, resistance, and flexibility training components of exercise medicine.

This book, *Exercise Medicine for the Frailty Syndrome*, is the opportunity to promote a well-rounded exercise medicine program and philosophy to improve the older adult's abilities and functional wellness before frailty concerns emerge. Also, the take-home message of the content is to highlight the importance of using an ASEP Board-Certified Exercise Physiologist to develop an individualized exercise medicine prescription when treating the elderly frail adult. The purpose of the intervention is to improve cardiovascular capacity, muscular strength and functional endurance, range of motion, and depression.

Ideally, the content should serve as a wake-up call to the academic exercise physiologists to work toward establishing a stronger relationship with exercise physiologists of the American Society of Exercise Physiologists. For certain, a credible career opportunity in health care will be recognized if there is support from the professors.

# PART I

# The Frailty Syndrome

## An Overview

# 1

# AGING AND THE FRAILTY SYNDROME

Although seldom a topic of discussion, frailty is a common geriatric syndrome. The primary factor associated with frailty is age-related disease pathologies. As individuals age, there is a deterioration and decrease in the physiologic function of specific molecular structures and cellular pathways. The result is often an increase in negative health outcomes that are the cornerstone of geriatric medicine and a decrease in the quality of living for the aging population.

From a healthcare perspective, there are numerous multifactorial etiologies that are linked to obesity and certain diseases that associate with the frailty syndrome. Researchers and healthcare professionals from different fields of work have provided an increased understanding of the biology of frailty. Its pathogenesis and clinical implications as well as the preventive and therapeutic interventions are better understood with respect to helping individuals at risk, those who have become frail from aging, different diseases, and/or medical conditions.

Frailty increases the vulnerability of individuals to increased dependency and/or early death compared to people without frailty (Morley et al. 2013). In adults over age 65, about 10% are frail and women, in particular, over age 80 are extremely likely to be frail. Weight loss in individuals over age 70 that is linked to chronic disease should be evaluated by a physician in anticipation of slowing or reversing the likelihood of falls and age-related physical disabilities due to frailty.

---

### BOX 1.1 WHAT IS FRAILTY?

While there is an international effort to define frailty, there is still no single definition or a commonly recognized assessment tool that is agreed upon by the research and/or medical community. The consensus on what frailty means is that it is a clinical syndrome (i.e., a collection of symptoms) that indicates increased susceptibility to various stressors leading to diminished strength, endurance, and physiological function that increase an individual's vulnerability for developing increased dependency and/or death.

—Morley JE, Vellas B, van Kan GA, et al. (2013). Frailty Consensus: A Call to Action. *Journal of the American Medical Directors Association*. 14;392–397.

---

DOI: 10.4324/9781003119920-2

Exercise physiologists have offered excellent leadership in the scientific study and application of exercise medicine (Boone 2016). Thus, given that an individual is diagnosed with frailty, the next healthcare professional to contact should be an ASEP Board-Certified Exercise Physiologist (ASEP 2018). The ASEP exercise physiologists have the scientific education and hands-on laboratory skills to help aging and frailty individuals by improving their muscle strength and endurance that decreases the tendency to experience fatigue and weight loss due to the decrease in lean muscle mass. The ASEP exercise medicine prescription helps to improve walking duration and speed, and decrease the tendency for and the effects of different chronic diseases.

The number of Americans who celebrate their 65th birthday is 10,000 every day. Longevity has reached a revolution level in the United States. This is both good and bad in that there is also a significant increase in the negative effects of aging and frailty. Interestingly, the aging nation is not aware that regular exercise can help reduce the severity of both conditions. As individuals age, it is important that they adhere to an exercise medicine routine if not daily, then every other day that involves aerobic exercise and resistance and flexibility training to build and maintain the functional integrity of the cardiorespiratory and musculoskeletal systems.

Exercise medicine is the answer to improving the health of geriatric patients and all others (including young and middle-aged adults) who are subject to a sedentary lifestyle. The downside of not doing so is multi-morbidity with a wide range of age-related diseases, clinical conditions, and diminished functional status. While exercise medicine can help prevent and/or treat the frailty syndrome of the age-associated decrease in physiologic function and reserve, the lack of exercise sets the stage for an increase in the susceptibility to stress, disability, risk of falls, hospitalization, and high rates of morbidity and mortality (Fried et al. 2001a).

Members of the public health community have increasingly become aware of their responsibility to better understand the bio-psycho-social difficulties that aging individuals may suffer from when living with the frailty syndrome. While the future may hold the possibility of intervening with pharmacological agents to prevent, treat, or reverse frailty, it is presently believed that the use of exercise medicine before the onset of an acute illness is the best approach to help ensure the aging person does not lose the in-built reserves of the multiple body systems. Otherwise, aging frail individuals with a loss of physiological reserve will experience an increase in acute illness, institutionalization, disease, and death (Fried et al. 2001b).

The following is a typical example of a series of adverse events in a 75-year-old woman with high blood pressure and congestive heart failure who lives with her husband. During the past year, she has become increasingly sensitive to the fact that there is no way to be active at home as usual due to her fatigue, headaches, and difficulty in breathing. Her husband is aware that his wife's health is getting worse. In fact, he has stepped up and helped his wife with her attempt to carry out the usual house cleaning. He did so due to her fatigue that was getting worse. She had stopped reaching out to her friends who live next door and around the block, and just recently shared with her husband that she had fallen and hurt her hip when he was at work. She also said to her husband that she felt the need to get some medical help. He agreed. Meantime, he is helping her when getting in and out of bed, taking a bath, and moving around in the house. After several weeks had past, the husband was convinced that his wife should see a medical doctor because she is not getting any better. In fact, the husband is beginning to realize that he will be her primary caregiver from this point forward.

As illustrated in this woman's case, frailty is marked by the decrease in physical function, muscle strength, and physiologic reserve. Cognitive impairment and depression were not part of her symptoms of frailty, although it is possible that they may occur as well (Ferrucci et al. 2004).

## Definitions of Frailty

Frailty is a combination of changes in the mind and body that often begins when aging adults are functioning reasonably well with minor changes in biological vulnerability and physiologic reserves. In time the individuals who are extremely frail experience failure in numerous systems throughout the body. These individuals are dependent on family, friends, and the medical system for help.

---

**BOX 1.2   THE FRAILTY SYNDROME.**

"A condition, seen particularly in older patients, characterized by low functional reserve, easy tiring, decreased libido, mood disturbance, accelerated osteoporosis, decreased muscle strength, and high susceptibility to disease. People with the frailty syndrome may take a sudden turn for the worse and die."

—*MedicineNet.* (2018). *Medical Definition of Frailty Syndrome* [Online]. www.Medicine. com/script/main/art.asp?articlekey=26356#osteoporosis_facts

---

Chin et al. (1999) compared three different definitions of frailty: (a) inactivity plus low energy intake; (b) inactivity plus weight loss; and (c) inactivity plus low body mass index. The subjects consisted of 450 independently living older males. They concluded that the combination of inactivity and weight loss was the most predictive of death and functional decline over a 3-year period. While their findings are interesting, it is commonly recognized that none of the definitions of frailty is considered the gold standard (Hamerman 1999).

Although there are varying definitions of frailty that are often generalized to the population under investigation, there is reasonably good agreement among the definitions. Regardless of the origin of the definition, it should address several qualifying points, such as included in the definition by the British Geriatrics Society (2016):

> Frailty is a distinctive health state related to the ageing process in which multiple body systems gradually lose their in-built reserves. Around 10 percent of people 65 years and older have frailty, rising to between a quarter and a half of the over 85 years. Older people living with frailty are at risk of adverse outcomes such as dramatic changes in their physical and mental wellbeing after an apparently minor event which challenges their health, such as an infection or new medication.

Although it may not be obvious at this point in the analysis of aging and the frailty syndrome, the scientific literature is in agreement that frailty can result in a functional decline to the point of producing serious adverse outcomes that include dependency, living in nursing homes, institutionalization, increase in healthcare spending, and early death. These points are highlighted in the following definition of frailty.

---

**BOX 1.3   THE INTERNATIONAL DEFINITION OF FRAILTY.**

"A medical syndrome with multiple causes and contributors that is characterized by diminished strength, endurance, and reduced physiologic function that increases an individual's vulnerability for developing increased dependency and/or death."

—Turpin, S. (2015). *What Is Frailty* [Online]. https://em3.org.uk/foamed/12/02/2015/ what-is-frailty

---

## Frailty Phenotype

In the absence of a medically agreed-upon definition of what is frailty, Fried et al. (2001b) defined frailty as meeting three of the five phenotypic criteria: (1) weakness (low grip strength), (2) low energy (self-reported exhaustion), (3) slowed walking speed (slowness), (4) low physical activity (low level of physical activity: males, 383 kcal·wk$^{-1}$ and females, 270 kcal·wk$^{-1}$), and (5) unintentional weight loss (>10 lbs within the past year).

A pre-frail state is recognized as an older individual who meets one or two of the phenotypic criteria. Older adults with none of the five criteria are classified as non-frail. Lee et al. (2017) concluded that screening for all five frailty markers, as required in the composite measures of the Fried frailty phenotype criteria, might be a major barrier to widespread frailty screening in the primary care setting. Therefore, they analyzed the five criteria as individual traits and as dual-factor combinations in 383 patients. They found that the dual-trait measure of gait speed with grip strength was accurate and more sensitive than individual traits.

When gait speed and handgrip strength were combined as a dual measure, the positive predictive value was 87.5%. Gait speed was calculated as the time (in seconds) to walk 4 meters (m) at a usual pace. The fastest time of two trials was recorded. Grip strength (in kilograms) was measured as the higher score of 2, 3-sec trials with each hand using a hand-held dynamometer.

Studenski et al. (2003) assess the ability of gait (i.e., walking) speed alone and a three-item lower extremity performance battery to predict 12-month rates of hospitalization, decline in health, and decline in function in primary care settings serving older adults. Gait speed alone predicted hospitalization; 41% (21/51) of slow walkers (gait speed 0.6 m·sec$^{-1}$) were hospitalized at least once, compared with 26% (70/266) of intermediate walkers (0.6–1.0 m·sec$^{-1}$) and 11% (15/136) of fast walkers (1.0 m·sec$^{-1}$). Given that frailty is primarily an older adult problem, the decrease in skeletal muscle strength and endurance associates with walking slower speeds.

To slow if not reverse the decrease in lean muscle mass, strength, and endurance, it is important that older adults engage in a combination of aerobic physical activity and low-intensity weight lifting exercises. The expectation is an improvement in functional capacity across several body systems that result in an increase in physiologic reserve, an increase in walking speeds, and a decrease in vulnerability to disease and death.

## Frailty Index

Contrary to the aforementioned researchers, Rockwood et al. (1999) and Mitnitski et al. (2001) used clinical information to identify adults at risk of poor outcomes. They developed the frailty index (FI) based on the impairments (or accumulated deficits) in cognitive status (i.e., psychosocial risk factors), mood, motivation, communication, mobility, balance, bowel and bladder function, activities of daily living, instrumental activities of daily living, nutrition, and social resources as well as common geriatric diseases and syndromes other than frailty (e.g., falls and delirium).

Interestingly, while the frailty index was found to be highly predictive of death or institutionalization, Chen et al. (2014) stated, "While the FI may have clinical utility in risk assessment and stratification, it is not clear if it adds significant value to comprehensive geriatric assessment. In addition, the FI does not attempt to distinguish frailty from disability or comorbidity." From a practical standpoint, Xue (2011) reported that the five-component phenotype is more appealing for use in clinical settings compared to the FI that typically contains 30 to 70 items.

## Frailty and Sarcopenia

Frailty is acknowledged as a multidimensional state of increased vulnerability due to the age-associated decline in physical, psychological (i.e., the decreased ability to cope with stressors), social, and environmental factors that influence the physiologic functions of a person (Gill et al. 2006). As a result of these factors either individually or collectively, frail adults suffer from a higher risk of adverse mind and body outcomes, physiologic impairments, and mortality. Frailty is also responsible for visits to the emergency department and/or hospitalizations, as well as decreasing the benefits of medical interventions and/or rendering complications and minimizing survival (Afilalo et al. 2010; Farhat et al. 2012).

It has become a major concern that a large proportion of frail elderly adults suffer from skeletal muscle wasting and weakness (i.e., sarcopenia) of which muscle strength is critical to walking without getting hurt and safely engaging in other physical and household activities necessary for independent living. The loss of lean muscle mass is the primary reason for a slow and unsteady gait that is a major pathology linked to feeling tired and/or exhausted with low levels of physical activity and a high risk of falling. As a result, frail adults often become dependent on family and friends to avoid hospitalization. If they end up in a hospital for a related health issue, they may not leave alive.

---

### BOX 1.4   WHAT HAPPENS TO FRAIL PATIENTS?

When frail patients are hospitalized, it is extremely important that they get out of bed several times a day to help prevent loss of muscle strength and power. Otherwise, the patients are likely to be exposed to an increase in the risk of thromboembolism, hypostatic pneumonia, and death.

There is also an important link between sarcopenia and various markers of poor quality of life, especially among certain chronic inflammatory conditions (Dodds & Sayer 2016). Thus, increasingly, persistent pro-inflammatory activity and dysregulation of the immune system are emerging as interesting factors in the genesis of sarcopenia and the frailty syndrome in general (Allen 2017). Frail people suffer from a constant low-grade inflammatory state due to the fact that the inflammatory signals get cut on to fight an infection or heal a wound but do not get turned off.

---

### BOX 1.5  SARCOPENIA IS A FREQUENT COMPONENT OF FRAILTY.

"Sarcopenia is not synonymous with frailty but, like other causes of muscle weakness, is an important contributing component of frailty in a large proportion of patients."

—Allen, SC. (2017). Systemic Inflammation in the Genesis of Frailty and Sarcopenia: An Overview of the Preventative and Therapeutic Role of Exercise and the Potential for Drug Treatments. *Geriatric.* 2;1–19.

---

While everyone experiences a decrease in the number and size of muscle fibers after 65 years of age, the older adult with sarcopenia is not the same as the effects of disuse atrophy. In fact, the changes are much worse in sarcopenia with a much higher loss of type 1 (slow-twitch) and type 2 (fast-twitch) fibers in aged muscles, which is why frail older adults are more likely to experience disabling falls and early death due to the muscle weakness, slow walking speed, and low levels of physical activity. They also experience greater difficulty in recovering from an illness or leaving a hospital after being admitted, given the decrease in physiologic reserves that leave them less able to adapt to acute illness or trauma.

### Physiologic Correlates of Frailty

Espinoza and Walston (2005) indicate that there are hypothesized interactions in specific physiologic systems and, in particular, the inflammatory and endocrine systems that influence changes in red blood cell production, skeletal muscle, blood clotting, and cellular metabolism in frail adults. They also indicate that these changes contribute to the symptoms experienced in frail older adults, as well as the changes resulting in an increased susceptibility to adverse health outcomes.

Morley et al. (2001) indicate that the endocrine system is involved in the changes in skeletal muscle mass and strength. In particular, the decrease in testosterone in the frail adult male is part of the reason for physical frailty. Similarly, in women, there is an age-related decrease in sex hormone levels with menopause (Poehlman et al. 1995) and, as frail adults age, there is a decrease in the growth hormone (Nass & Thorner 2002), which does not happen in non-frail older adults. Therefore, given that the growth hormone is important in the stimulation of the sex hormone dehydroepiandrosterone sulfate and the insulin-like growth factor-1 (IGF-1, a messenger molecule that is stimulated by the growth hormone) (Leng et al. 2004), frail older adults have lower levels of the sex hormone.

While there are other hormones that help to prevent the loss of muscle strength and may also be important in understanding and treating frailty (Montero-Odasso & Duque 2005), Espinoza and Walston (2005) indicate that it is necessary to do more research to understand the connections. In particular, adults with the frailty syndrome should undergo a more in-depth assessment of the immune system. A starting point is to evaluate adults aged 70 years and older with an unintentional weight loss (Fried et al. 2001b) in association with a chronic illness. The abundance of immune compounds renders a person extremely weak if not fatigued and unable to carry out daily activities.

Adult frailty is the result of a state of ongoing systemic inflammation due to the unrelenting immune activation. That is why a person's elevated levels of the pro-inflammatory cytokine interleukin-6 (IL-6) and C-reactive protein are recognized as a predictor of the risk of becoming frail (Leng et al. 2002; Walston et al. 2002), as well as an increase in morbidity and mortality in older adults (De et al. 2006). Li et al. (2011) indicate that elevated IL-6 levels are associated with a decrease in muscle strength and power that result in a slow walking speed, which are two components of the frailty syndrome. In addition, Ershler (2003) indicates that IL-6 may result in anemia by interfering with normal iron metabolism or directly by inhibiting the production of erythropoietin.

---

## BOX 1.6   THE INFLAMMATORY IL-6 MARKER IN FRAILTY.

Age-related increases in IL-6 levels are associated with atherosclerosis, osteoporosis, and sarcopenia, and with functional decline, disability, and all-cause mortality in older adults.

—Li, H, et al. (2011). Frailty, Inflammation, and Immunity. *Aging and Disease*. 2;466–473.

---

Walston et al. (2002) reported findings supporting the hypothesis that there is a specific physiologic basis for the geriatric syndrome of frailty. They concluded that it is characterized in part by not only increased inflammation but also elevated markers of ongoing clotting activity (specifically, factor VIII, fibrinogen, and D dimer). Moreover, these physiological differences persisted even when the individuals with diabetes and cardiovascular disease were excluded and after adjustment for age, sex, and race.

## Final Thoughts

Kinsella et al. (2005) indicate that globally, the proportion of adults aged 65 years and older is growing, from 461 million people in 2004 to a projected 2 billion by 2050. The aging population will manifest physical frailty and sarcopenia, both of which are associated with adverse health-related problems (Clegg et al. 2013). To date, there are several definitions of frailty, but no consensus has been reached on the definitions. In general, it is apparent that frailty is a medical syndrome with numerous causes that decrease muscle strength in particular and physiological function in general. The end result is an increase in the older adults' vulnerability to dependency and/or death.

It is interesting that to some extent the underlying health issues of frailty are very similar to the outcomes associated with sarcopenia. Hence, frail older adults are recognized by signs and symptoms that include loss of skeletal muscle mass, strength, and weakness, weight loss, fatigue, decrease in physical activity, slow movements and/or unsteady gait, increase in likelihood of falls, and loss of autonomy. In an attempt to better conceptualize frailty, multiple frailty scales have been researched and used. Compared to the Frailty Index, the Fried Frailty Phenotype measure of gait speed and grip strength is widely used to identify older adults with high risk of adverse functional impairment, adverse health outcomes, and mortality. As a progressive disorder involving the loss of muscle mass, it is a primary concern because it plays an important etiologic role in the frailty process. Also, it is associated with an increase in the risk of disability, all-cause mortality, and higher healthcare costs. Either directly or indirectly, the older adults' chronic inflammatory state is marked by an increase in IL-6 levels than non-frail controls of similar age.

---

**BOX 1.7   MOLECULAR AND CELLULAR INFLAMMATORY MARKERS IN FRAILTY.**

Interleukin 6 (IL-6) is a pro-inflammatory cytokine that is increased in the circulation of older adults. Aside from being associated with atherosclerosis and osteoporosis in older adults, increased IL-6 levels are also associated with lower muscle mass and strength in frail older adults. Leng et al. (2002) presented evidence that supports the relationship of the molecular inflammatory marker with frailty in a pilot study in which community-dwelling frail older adults had significantly higher IL-6 levels than non-frail controls of similar age.

—Leng, S, Chaves, P, Koenig, K, Walston, J. (2002). Serum Interleukin-6 and Hemoglobin as Physiological Correlates in the Geriatric Syndrome of Frailty: A Pilot Study. *Journal of the American Geriatric Society.* 50;1268–1271.

---

## References

Afilalo, J, Eisenberg, MJ, Morin, JF, et al. (2010). Gait Speed as an Incremental Predictor of Mortality and Major Morbidity in Elderly Patients Undergoing Cardiac Surgery. *Journal of the American College of Cardiology.* 56;1668–1676.

Allen, SC. (2017). Systemic Inflammation in the Genesis of Frailty and Sarcopenia: An Overview of the Preventative and Therapeutic Role of Exercise and the Potential for Drug Treatments. *Geriatric.* 2;1–19.

*American Society of Exercise Physiologists.* (2018). *Board Certified Exercise Physiologists* [Online]. www.asep.org/epc-online/epc-missionpurpose/

*BGS Guideline.* (2016). Fit for Frailty [Online]. www.bgs.org.uk/index.php/fit-for-frailty

Boone, T. (2016). *ASEP's Exercise Medicine Text for Exercise Physiologists.* Beijing, China: Bentham Science Publishers.

British Geriatrics Society. (2016). *What Is Frailty?* London: British Geriatrics Society. http://www.bgs.org.uk/frailty-explained/resources/campaigns/fit-for-frailty/frailty-what-is-it

Chen, X, Mao, G, Leng, SX. (2014). Frailty Syndrome: An Overview. *Clinical Interventions in Aging.* 9;433–441.

Chin, A, Paw, MJ, Dekker, JM, et al. (1999). How to Select a Frail Elderly Population? A Comparison of Three Working Definitions. *Journal of Clinical Epidemiology.* 52;1015–1021.

Clegg, A, Young, J, Lliffe, S, et al. (2013). Frailty in Elderly People. *Lancet.* 381;752–762.

De, MM, Franceschi, C, Monti, D, et al. (2006). Inflammation Markers Predicting Frailty and Mortality in the Elderly. *Experimental and Molecular Pathology.* 80;219–227.

Dodds, RM, Sayer, AA. (2016). Sarcopenia, Frailty and Mortality: The Evidence Is Growing. *Age Ageing.* 45;570–571.

Ershler, WB. (2003). Biological Interactions of Aging and Anemia: A Focus on Cytokines. *Journal of the American Geriatric Society.* 51;18–21.

Espinoza, S, Walston, JD. (2005). Frailty in Older Adults: Insights and Interventions. *Cleveland Clinic Journal of Medicine.* 72;1105–1112.

Farhat, JS, Velanovich, V, Falvo, AJ, et al. (2012). Are the Frail Destined to Fail? Frailty Index as a Predictor of Surgical Morbidity and Mortality in the Elderly. *Journal of Trauma Acute Care Surgery.* 72;1526–1530.

Ferrucci, L, Guralnik, JM, Studenski, S, et al. (2004). Designing Randomized, Controlled Trials Aimed at Preventing or Delaying Functional Decline and Disability in Frail, Older Persons: A Consensus Report. *Journal of American Geriatric Society.* 52;625–634.

Fried, LP, Tangen, CM, Walston, J, et al. (2001a). Cardiovascular Health Study Collaborative Research Group. Frailty in Older Adults: Evidence for a Phenotype. *Journal of Gerontology: Medical Sciences.* 56A;146–156.

Fried, LP, Tangen, CM, Walston, J, et al. (2001b). Frailty in Older Adults: Evidence for a Phenotype. *Journal of Gerontology: Biological Sciences and Medical Sciences.* 56(3);146–156.

Gill, TM, Gahbauer, EA, Allore, HG, Han, L. (2006). Transitions between Frailty States Among Community-Living Older Persons. *Archives of Internal Medicine.* 4;418–423.

Hamerman, D. (1999). Toward an Understanding of Frailty. *Annals of Internal Medicine.* 130;945–950.

Kinsella, KG, Phillips, DR. (2005). *Global Aging: The Challenge of Success.* Washington, DC: Population Reference Bureau.

Lee, L, Patel, T, Costa, A, et al. (2017). Screening for Frailty in Primary Care: Accuracy of Gait Speed and Hand-Grip Strength. *Canadian Family Physician.* 63;e51–e57.

Leng, SX, Cappola, AR, Andersen, RE, et al. (2004). Serum Levels of Insulin-Like Growth Factor 1 (IGF-1) and Dehydroepiandrosterone Sulfate (DHEA-5), and Their Relationships With Serum Interleukin-6, in the Geriatric Syndrome of Frailty. *Aging Clinical and Experimental Research.* 16;153–157.

Leng, SX, Chaves, P, Koenig, K, Walston, J. (2002). Serum Interleukin-6 and Hemoglobin as Physiological Correlates in the Geriatric Syndrome of Frailty: A Pilot Study. *Journal of the American Geriatric Society.* 50;1268–1271.

Li, H, Manwani, B, Leng, SX. (2011). Frailty, Inflammation, and Immunity. *Aging and Disease.* 2;466–473.

Mitnitski, AB, Mogilner, AJ, Rockwood, K. (2001). Accumulation of Deficits as a Proxy Measure of Aging. *The Scientific World.* 1;323–336.

Montero-Odasso, M, Duque, G. (2005). Vitamin D in the Aging Musculoskeletal System: An Authentic Strength Preserving Hormone. *Molecular Aspects of Medicine.* 26;203–219.

Morley, JE, Baumgartner, RN, Roubenoff, R, et al. (2001). Sarcopenia. *Journal of Laboratory and Clinical Medicine.* 137;231–243.

Morley, JE, Vellas B, van Kan GA, et al. (2013). Frailty Consensus: A Call to Action. *Journal of the American Medical Directors Association.* 14;392–397.

Nass, R, Thorner, MO. (2002). Impact of the GH-Cortisol Ratio on the Age-Dependent Changes in Body Composition. *Growth Hormone IGF Research.* 12;147–161.

Poehlman, ET, Toth, MJ, Fishman, PS, et al. (1995). Sarcopenia in Aging Humans: The Impact of Menopause and Disease. *Journal of Gerontology: Biological Sciences and Medical Sciences.* 50;73–77.

Rockwood, K, Stadnyk, K, MacKnight, C, et al. (1999). A Brief Clinical Instrument to Classify Frailty in Elderly People. *Lancet.* 353;205–206.

Studenski, S, Perera, S, Wallace, D, et al. (2003). Physical Performance Measures in the Clinical Setting. *Journal of the American Geriatrics Society.* 51;314–322.

Walston, J, McBurnie, MA, Newman, A, et al. (2002). Frailty and Activation of the Inflammation and Coagulation Systems With and Without Clinical Morbidities: Results from the Cardiovascular Health Study. *Archives of Internal Medicine.* 162;2333–2341.

Xue, Q-L. (2011). The Frailty Syndrome: Definition and Natural History. *Clinics in Geriatric Medicine.* 27;1–15.

# 2

# FRAILTY, OBESITY, NUTRITION, AND COGNITIVE STATUS

To develop a better understanding of frailty as a geriatric syndrome, it is important to acknowledge different factors that contribute to the pathogenesis of frailty. For example, what is aging? What are the changes at the cellular level in older people, particularly with regard to systemic responses to stressors? What are the drivers and the current cornerstones of interventions for optimal aging? Can frail older adults also be obese? Since frailty is a major predictor of comorbidities and mortality, what is the role of nutrition, protein supplementation, essential amino acid supplementation, beta-hydroxy-beta-methylbutyrate (HMB), vitamin D, and different exercise modalities in minimizing the adverse changes that occur with frailty and sarcopenia with the aim of improving mind and body health?

## Population, Aging, and Disease

It is not a good idea to turn a blind eye to the aging process. According to Puett (2018), "The number of people 65 and older in the United States is approximately 15%, and in less than 15 years, 1 in 5 Americans (20%) will fall into this category." The growth in the number of older adults in the United States and throughout the world is unprecedented. It is anticipated that by 2030 Americans aged 65 or older will be about 72 million (Wan et al. 2005) and close to 89 million by 2050, which is more than twice the number of older adults in the United States in 2010 (US Census Bureau).

Americans are living into their seventies, eighties, and nineties. Since 2011, and each day for the next 20 years, ~10,000 adults will celebrate their 65th birthday (Pew Research Center). This is a good thing, right? Yes, of course, it is but there are challenges to society as more adults get older. Aside from the personal challenges with aging, there are profound effects on our nation's public health and well-being, social services, and healthcare systems due to chronic conditions (CDC 2013).

With regard to the aging adults with chronic disease, in particular, a tremendous burden is placed on Medicare. In fact, almost all Medicare spending is on behalf of older adults with at least one chronic disease. Hoffman and Rice (1996) indicate that by 2020 the United States will spend ~$685 billion a year in direct medical costs for persons with chronic diseases, and by 2050, it will increase to ~$906 billion. Despite the increased information about physical

DOI: 10.4324/9781003119920-3

frailty and sarcopenia, it is clear that the prevalence and incidence of chronic disease are only going to get worse. The average 75-year-old suffers from three chronic diseases and takes five prescription medications (Merck Institute of Aging and Health 2004).

---

### BOX 2.1  AGING AND CHRONIC DISEASES.

*During the 20th century, the population of Americans 85 years of age and older increased from just over 100,000 to 4.2 million.*

—Federal Interagency Forum on Aging-Related Statistics 2004, *Older Americans.*

*About 80% of the aging population has one or more chronic diseases such as heart disease, cancer, stroke, chronic obstructive pulmonary disease, and diabetes.*

—Goldman, DP, Cutler, D, Shang, B, Joyce, G. (2005). *The Value of Elderly Disease Prevention.* Washington, DC: Centers for Medicare and Medicaid Services.

---

## Aging and Frailty

To better understand the concept of frailty as a geriatric syndrome, it is important to know the difference between normal age-related changes and frailty. Aging is a decrease in maintaining specific molecular structures and pathways, a decrease in adaptability to stressors, a loss of homeostasis, and a failure of biologic systems to maintain functional capacity. While it is true that individuals vary greatly in the onset and progression of aging, it is inevitable that everyone will get older. One out of every eight people (i.e., roughly 12% of the population) is an older person and the number of people 100 years of age and older increased by 36% between 1900 and 2003 (Administration on Aging 2004).

Adults age along a continuum of aging well without frailty and/or disability or they experience some or many of the multidimensional factors that characterize the frailty syndrome. Hence, along the continuum an adult male may display a strong reserve, freedom from disability, independent functioning, and increased resistance to stressors or he may be living with a decreased reserve and diminished ability to adapt physically and mentally. While aging often requires some clinical care, it is not true that all aging individuals have poor health and/or fitness or even a chronic disease. However, it is true that aging adults who are frail more often than not have clinical and/or laboratory biomarkers that require treatment.

---

### BOX 2.2  SUCCESSFUL AGING.

The term "successful aging" was first coined six decades ago. Adults who age successfully are functionally independent with no physical issues and/or disabilities. They demonstrate high cognitive and physical functioning. However, future research findings will probably suggest the likelihood of a high prevalence of aging adults who fall in the overlap zone between the two paradigms. This isn't a problem since all adults, regardless of age, need to adhere to an exercise medicine prescription.

—Havighurst, R. (1961). Successful Aging. *Gerontologist.* 1;8–13.

---

Successful aging is associated with a decreased risk for poor health outcomes, including falls, disability, hospitalization, and mortality. Adults who are aware of the importance of regular exercise represent the individuals who are not likely to live with age-related decreases in strength and tolerance for physical exertion.

Understandably, it is critical that high-risk subsets of older adults who are living with the clinical manifestations of frailty have the opportunity to participate in an exercise medicine program supervised by qualified healthcare professional (such as an ASEP Board-Certified Exercise Physiologist) to help avoid the increased risk of poor health outcomes. An individualized adult-specific resistance training (RT) program can help increase lean muscle mass and, therefore, slow the exacerbating issues that come with sarcopenia. In particular, RT can bring about an increase in muscle strength to help ensure a higher level of energy, faster walking speed, and a higher level of physical activity.

---

**BOX 2.3   THE BENEFITS OF PROGRESSIVE RESISTANCE TRAINING PROGRAM FOR FRAILTY.**

Qian-Li Xue stated, "Frailty is a clinical syndrome in older adults that can result in disability, diseases, physical and cognitive impairments, psychosocial risk factors, and geriatric syndromes (e.g., falls, delirium, and urinary incontinence)."

—Xue, Qian-Li. (2011). The Frailty Syndrome: Definition and Natural History. *Clinical Geriatric Medicine*. 27;1–15.

---

Building on this conceptual framework laid out by Dr. Xue is it not understandable that carefully helping an older adult client who has been diagnosed as frail is extremely likely by way of a client-specific RT exercise medicine prescription. This point of view is not rocket science! It makes sense that sarcopenia can be reversed by a systematic RT program that consists of 2 to 3 d·wk$^{-1}$ of low intensity that allows for the execution of 8 to 10 exercises using 1 to 3 sets per exercise with 8 to 12 repetitions. The selection of exercises should produce an increase in the lean muscle mass and strength of the upper and lower extremities. The benefits are huge. The increase in upper and lower muscle strength will help decrease the chances of physical disability, falls, and fractures. Mental health will improve due to a better physical appearance.

The purpose of the RT program as part of a multifaceted (i.e., aerobics training and nutritional information) exercise medicine prescription is to produce improvement in the age-related physiologic reserve and function across multiple systems. When done correctly, the result is a decrease in the frailty severity that allows the client to better cope with the mental and physical stressors experienced in daily life. Having made this point, however, it is very likely that aging and pathologies share similar if not the same common mechanisms (Franceschi et al. 2018).

## Obesity and Frailty

Not only being obese (BMI of 30 kg·m$^{-2}$ or more) is linked to a decrease in quality of life and an increase in mortality but it also contributes to coronary heart disease (Bales & Buhr 2008), fatal and nonfatal myocardial infarctions (Harris et al. 1997), and mortality from cardiovascular disease (Dey & Lissner 2003). As of a 2012 paper by Mathus-Vliegen, more than 33% of adults over age 60 in the United States are obese. This is a problem on many different levels since obesity leads to a decrease in aerobic capacity, which has a negative effect on performing physical daily tasks (Gates et al. 2008). Moreover, excessive adiposity increases the risk of personal injury (Schmier et al. 2006).

The excess of stores in the adipose tissue increases oxidative stress. During over-nutrition, adipocytes release more reactive oxygen species (ROS) in accordance with the following steps: First, as a result of overeating, the adipocytes release more ROS and pro-inflammatory cytokines that lead to a continuous condition of "simmering" inflammation. Second, when the obesity-driven inflammatory cascade is coupled with age-related inflammation, the increased catabolism and blunted anabolism are detrimental to the muscular system (Ershler 2007).

Third, the increased catabolism along with the muscle damage from the elevated ROS results in a decrease in the adult's muscle mass and strength. Fourth, the overall effect is muscle weakness and slow activation of the muscles that are easy to exhaust. Fifth, the increase in difficulty in using the muscles contributes to the difficulty in human movement necessary to keep from being obese (Starr et al. 2014).

Lipid deposition in skeletal muscle is an aging and obesity problem, given that the muscular system is responsible for physical movement. Morphological changes that result from the increase in lipid accumulation within the muscle fibers decrease muscle density that creates a loss of muscle strength separate from the changes in the lean muscle mass (Goodpaster et al. 2000; Moro et al. 2009; Goodpaster et al. 2001). Ultimately, the lipid that infiltrates the muscle tissue leads to an increase in the vulnerability of adults 65 years of age or older to a wide range of adverse health outcomes linked to an increase in mortality.

---

**BOX 2.4   THE NEGATIVE EFFECT OF LIPID FILTRATION.**

Jensen and Hsiao (2010) indicate that the loss of muscle strength in aging obese adults is due more so to the decrease in muscle quality than to the decrease in skeletal muscle mass, which is a good indication of the negative effect of lipid infiltration that impairs muscle function.

—Jensen, GL, Hsiao, PY. (2010). Obesity in Older Adults: Relationship to Functional-Limitation. *Current Opinion in Clinical Nutrition and Metabolic Care.* 13(1);46–51.

---

The logical approach to dealing with obesity and frailty is to prevent either from happening. If the client is already showing signs of either or both conditions, then the logical corrective action is to get the older adult to change his or her lifestyle to avoid physical and/or mental suffering, disability, and dependence. The goal is to help the client to stay active and therefore healthy. This means that adherence to an exercise medicine prescription is imperative. If successful in doing so, the aging adult should live longer with fewer biomedical health issues.

Strangely enough, considerable education in society is presently required along with the motivation to repair and improve their bodies to realize a long and healthy lifespan. Society will come to understand the importance of exercise medicine as a multicomponent exercise intervention to prevent falls and increase mobility and muscle strength.

ASEP Board-Certified Exercise Physiologists can help guide and supervise aging adults with diverse components of the frailty syndrome. With the improvement in frailty, the elderly adults will experience less often the need to be institutionalized or hospitalized due to improved physical functions and quality of life (de Labra et al. 2015). But, until society recognizes that frailty and disability are on the rise in the United States, it is crucial that society understands the negative effects of frailty in aging adults. The decrease in functional status along with the consequences of different chronic conditions leave millions of older adults who are subject to falls, fractures, hospitalization, loss of mobility, institutionalization, and death.

## Frailty, Disability, and Healthcare Costs

Frailty is a geriatric syndrome that not only is linked to an increase in morbidity and mortality but many aging adults who are frail also live with disability and the need for help with daily activities. No doubt there are many frail adults who have functional difficulties with many daily activities, and yet they are not receiving help. If they were identified early during their elderly years, then it is possible to prevent them from becoming frail or at least slow down the process to help improve their quality of life (such as when they walk a short distance, climb stairs, and/or feel they have enough energy to complete other daily activities).

---

**BOX 2.5  FRAILTY, DISABILITY, AND HEALTHCARE COST.**

"Disability is defined as difficulty or dependency in carrying out activities essential to independent living, including essential roles, tasks needed for self-care and living independently in a house, and desired activities important to one's quality of life."

—Fried, LP, Ferrucci, L, Darer, J, et al. (2004). Untangling the Concepts of Disability, Frailty, and Comorbidity: Implications for Improved Targeting and Care. *Journal of Gerontology.* 59(3);255–263.

In 2000, 1.5 million frail adults were institutionalized in the United States. Thirty-three percent of the aging adults were admitted to long-term healthcare facilities due to their decreased mobility at a cost of billions of healthcare dollars.

—Janssen et al. (2004). The Healthcare Costs of Sarcopenia in the United States. *Journal of the American Geriatric Society.* 52;80–85.

---

The growing population of frail and older adults with multiple chronic conditions or comorbidity (Hoffman et al. 1996) or those who are disabled is a serious medical entity (Pope & Tarlov 1991) as is true with most physical disabilities. Fried et al. (2004) said, "Disability is defined as difficulty or dependency in carrying out activities essential to independent living, including essential roles, tasks needed for self-care and living independently in a house, and desired activities important to one's quality of life." The end result is usually the adult living in a nursing home. Thus, ultimately, disability in late life (such as skeletal muscle weakness and decrease in physical activity tolerance) is associated with an increase in high healthcare costs due to the need for long-term care and hospitalization (Fried & Guralnik 1997; Fried et al. 1998).

Disability is not something to be taken lightly. Older adults who are disabled are at risk of social isolation, comorbid diseases, dependency, and the need for long-term health care and intervention (Fried et al. 2004). Guralnik et al. (1995) researched and reported on these points in a representative sample of moderately to severely disabled community-dwelling women aged 65 to 101 years. Seventy-four percent (742) of the 1,002 subjects in their study reported difficulty walking two to three blocks.

Fifteen percent (150) of the subjects were homebound and 1,146% (461) lived alone. Forty-five percent (451) of the subjects had difficulty bathing, 21% (210) had difficulty dressing themselves, and 37% (371) had trouble with blurred vision. Twenty-eight percent (281) of the women identified as being frail. They had an average of 4.3 chronic diseases. Fried et al. (2004) indicated that this population of women is at a high risk of social isolation, which highlights the complexity of dealing with healthcare issues (i.e., preventing further frailty, physiologic decline, decrements in mobility, and further loss of independence).

Without the opportunity for preventive and/or corrective action, Fried et al. (2004) pointed out that the existence of frailty, disability and/or functional limitation, and comorbidity singly or collectively increases both the need and costs for health care. Also, when two or more of these conditions exist at the same time, there is the expectation of a significant additive healthcare costs. Clearly, this is an important concern since two or more chronic conditions with disability and functional limitation resulted in a total inpatient and medication expenditure costs of $4,865 compared to adults without a disability and functional limitation that resulted in a total inpatient and medication expenditure costs of $316.

The presence of comorbidity markedly increases with aging because it is associated with an increase in chronic diseases. Hoffman et al. (1996) and Adams et al. (1999) reported that after 65 years of age, 48% of the community-dwelling adults in the United States were arthritic, 36% were hypertensive, 27% were diagnosed with heart disease, 10% were diabetic, and 6% had a stroke. Although the findings by Guralnik et al. (1989) are from the 1980s (i.e., 40 years ago), they are helpful in understanding the concerns of elderly adults. For example, 35.3% of the population in the United States between 65 and 79 years of age reported two or more diseases. But, when the adults reached 80 years of age and older, the percentage increased to 70.2%, which is also why the Medicare claims for the presence of two diseases are linked to higher expenditures (Anderson 2002).

This is a financial concern, given that the American Medical Association has stated that 40% of the adults who are 80 years of age or older are frail (Council on Scientific Affairs 1990). Also, as Gabrel (2000) has pointed out, the majority of the 1.6 million elderly nursing home residents in the United States suffer from the physiologic stressors that result from the decrease in physiologic reserves. The frail adults and the disabled older adults are also at risk of progressive weakness, weight loss, social isolation due to sensory and mobility impairments, and the need for medical care for acute illness or injury, comorbid diseases, and depression that increase their healthcare cost. The overall medical and medication costs that result from being an older frail adult with a disability and multiple chronic diseases are likely to be in the range of four or five times greater than the costs of frailty or disability without a disease condition.

---

### BOX 2.6  FRAILTY AND PHYSICAL DISABILITY.

Independent of comorbid diseases, the clinical observations of a decrease in muscle mass and strength, bodyweight, and physical endurance have a negative effect on an older frail adult's ability to balance, to be mobile, and to be able to move at a different gait speed. As a result, adults aged 65 years and older with evidence of being frail are an independent cause of physical disability.

---

## Frailty, Exercise, and Nutrition

Individuals over the age of 80 represent the fastest-growing elderly adult age group in the United States (Topinkova 2008). Many of the aging adults are living with an increase in vulnerability to stressors that individually and/or collectively result in a decrease in bodyweight, a decrease in lean muscle mass, an increase in muscle weakness and overall fatigue, a decrease in physical activity, a significantly greater limitation in walking, and an increase in disability associated with mobility tasks. Compared to non-frail older adults, frail older adults are seven times more likely to be admitted to a hospital with more visits to different physicians (Experton et al. 1996).

Not only are there nutritional issues and concerns with aging but obesity can also increase the age-related decrease in physiologic function and different reasons for frailty in aging adults. Villareal et al. (2006) highlighted this point in their research in which they exercised frail obese older adults 3 times·wk$^{-1}$ for 6 months. Compared with the control group, fat mass decreased while peak oxygen consumption (VO$_2$ peak), muscle strength, walking speed, and one-leg limb stance time increased in the frail obese older adults. Although the decrease in fat mass is a good finding, there is the concern that losing weight (i.e., if it involves muscle mass, too) can have an adverse influence on health status even with an increase in muscle strength. Hence, "weight loss" is not equivalent to being healthy if it is a combination of losing fat and muscle tissue.

With growing older, it is important that physical activity (primarily in the form of regular exercise) is increased while also consuming a good nutritional diet, given the association between micronutrients and frailty. Both are important in reducing the risk of chronic diseases (Fairfield & Fletcher 2002), osteoporotic fractures (Rizzoli 2010), peripheral arterial disease (Lane et al. 2008), and frailty (Michelon et al. 2006). In particular, Bartali et al. (2006) reported that a low intake of vitamins D, E, and C, and folate was related to frailty independent of energy consumption. As well, Michelon et al. (2006) reported that the age-adjusted odds ratios of being frail were higher for older women with lower levels of micronutrients, such as serum total carotenoids, α-tocopherol, 25-hydroxyvitamin D, and vitamin B$_6$.

Kobayashi et al. (2013) found that a higher intake of total protein was significantly associated with a lower prevalence of frailty among older Japanese women. Their findings were true regardless of whether the protein source was fish, shellfish, meat, eggs, cereals, potatoes, fruits, or vegetables. Their findings also indicated the type of amino acids that composed the protein did matter in the prevention of frailty. The findings also highlight that frailty is a late-life syndrome that is the result of a number of different problems associated with aging that is likely to get much worse throughout the world.

---

**BOX 2.7 THE AGING OF THE WORLD POPULATION.**

According to current findings, it is estimated that the number of people globally who are aged 60 years or over will increase from 901 million to 1.4 billion between 2015 and 2030 and that the number will increase to nearly 2.1 billion by 2050.

—*United Nations*. (2015). *World Population Ageing 2015* [Online]. www.un.Org/en/development/desa/population/publications/pdf/ageing/WPA 2015_Report.pdf

---

The bottom line is that the nutritional status of middle-aged adults is part of not only physical frailty but also cognitive frailty in older adults. Thus, even if research does not identify a specific type of food or supplement that precipitates physical frailty and/or cognitive impairment, poor nutrition and overeating in middle age have been associated with cognitive decline (Dominguez & Barbagallo 2017).

## Frailty, Impairments, and Costs

Whether the cause of physical and/or cognitive frailty is an age factor or the result of multiple factors, Guyonnet et al. (2015) stated that it can be treated by correcting the dysregulated energetics involving the physiological and molecular pathways. However, if left untreated the older frail adult can experience several negative considerations (e.g., inflammation, sarcopenia, decreased heart rate variability, altered insulin resistance, altered clotting processes, anemia, micronutrient deficiencies, and altered hormone levels). When these physiological impairments are interpreted as clinical characteristics, it isn't difficult to understand that frailty is linked to longer than usual hospital stays and increased mortality in hospitalized patients (Khandelwal et al. 2012).

Being overweight, obese, and living with specific lifestyle-related factors are linked to health problems and markers of pre-frailty and frailty consequences just as they are to late-life cognitive impairment and decline (Solfrizzi et al. 2012). This is also the case when older adults consume a low dietary intake of protein (Blaum et al. 2005) and other micro- and macronutrients. Thus, it should be obvious that healthcare professionals are responsible for identifying the steps to slow the burdens associated with the frailty process (Fairhall et al. 2011). They should be involved in the prevention of frailty altogether and/or the decrease in adverse outcomes to improve the aging adults' quality of life, which may be more promising with the prescription of multi-domain interventions.

---

**BOX 2.8 THE OPTIMAL TYPE OF EXERCISE INTERVENTION.**

Dedeyne et al. (2017) indicate that there is limited but promising data supporting a combination of exercise and nutritional intervention (with a high protein intake) versus just an exercise intervention or just a nutrition intervention may be the better approach to improve frailty status.

> The same thinking would be true for targeting two or more of the following domains (e.g., pharmacological and hormonal or nutritional and cognitive therapy). But, with regard to exercise physiology, it is always important to remember that exercise is the key to health and longevity.

Mezey and Fulmer (1998) reported that frail older adults have a higher frequency of primary care visits, consume 50% of all hospital care, use over 80% of the home care services, and occupy 90% of all nursing home beds in the United States. Frail older adults obviously require an abundance of health services to deal with their acute and chronic illnesses and/or injuries. The particular array of services for frail individuals depends on their specific needs (such as cognitive decline) and numerous other concerns at a high cost. As an example, Knickman and Snell (2002) indicated that older adults can expect to spend out of pocket around $90,000, which is an estimate of $44,000 for long-term care, $18,000 for private insurance, $16,000 for medical care not paid by Medicare or private insurance, and $12,000 for prescription drugs.

There are other financial concerns as well. According to Dyeson et al. (1999), numerous items that are required by older adults to live a functionally independent lifestyle are not paid for by Medicare. For example, Medicare does pay for dental care that might include oral exams, cleanings, fillings, bridges, and/or crowns, eyeglasses and contact lenses, dentures, foot care, many medications, and hearing aids or exams. The impact of frailty and the market value of this care will produce (along with the increase in prevalence of osteoporosis, diabetes, glaucoma, cataracts, heart disease, cancer, arthritis, and obesity) an increased percentage of older adults who will be heavily dependent on mind and body healthcare services.

## Cognitive Frailty

In the context of aging, physical frailty is an accepted term. However, as pointed out by Woods et al. (2013), the term cognitive frailty is not that well understood. The concept of cognitive frailty was proposed in 2006 by Panza et al. (2015). A general consensus is that cognitive frailty refers to cognitive impairments that are linked to the aging process. Cognitive frailty is not meant to be acknowledged the same as some pre-existing brain disorders or dementia (Kelaiditi et al. 2013). Cognitive frailty is the loss of an individual's ability to resist impairments at the cognitive level. Physiological function of the brain is decreased. The adult's cognitive reserve is less than what it was prior to the influence of the aging process and/or cognitive disturbances secondary to chronic conditions such as diabetes and cardiovascular disease (Cohen et al. 2009).

Dynapenia (i.e., slowness and/or weakness) is associated with physical pre-frailty and frailty state as well as with cognitive frailty. The slowness and/or weakness of the two frailty types are linked to the decrease in gray matter in the cerebellum in addition to the age-related cognitive impairment. Thus, frail persons with cognitive impairment are more likely to develop disability in activities of daily living (ADLs). Also, it is generally the consensus that the frailty syndrome and cognitive frailty are associated with an increased risk of falls, disability, hospitalization, and death.

---

### BOX 2.9  A WORKING DEFINITION OF COGNITIVE FRAILTY.

Cognitive frailty is defined as the presence of cognitive deficits in physically frail older persons without dementia. This subtype of frailty is deemed important, as it may represent a prodromal phase for neurodegenerative diseases and is potentially a suitable target for early intervention.

—Fougere, B, et al. (2017). Cognitive Frailty: Mechanisms, Tools to Measure, Prevention and Controversy. *Clinics in Geriatric Medicine*. 33;339—355.

---

## Final Thoughts

The number of older adults throughout the world has increased substantially in recent years, and it is projected to accelerate in the coming decades. For example, in 2014, 14.5% (46.3 million) of the population in the United States was aged 65 or older. By 2060, it is expected to reach 23.5% (98 million) (Colby & Ortman 2014). Professionals, such as the ASEP Board-Certified Exercise Physiologists, as well as paid and unpaid caregivers must be prepared to improve the care of these adults (Institute of Medicine 2008).

As healthcare professionals, exercise physiologists with the ASEP education and laboratory training in exercise physiology are in an excellent position to help the elderly frail adults with their disability issues that associate with sarcopenia, obesity, and poor nutrition. Their supervision of the adults' exercise medicine program is also expected to help with cognitive issues given that regular exercise plays an important role in decreasing stress and depression.

With the influence of exercise medicine, it is anticipated that the frequency of the primary care visits by frail older adults will decrease. More elderly adults should be physically better prepared to stay in their homes instead of occupying nursing beds or living in other community dwellings. They will experience an increase in their reserve capacity of multiple body systems and feel physically stronger.

## References

Adams, PF, Hendershot, GE, Marano, MA. (1999). Current Estimates from the National Health Interview Survey, United States, 1966. *Vital and Health Statistics, Series 10, No. 200*. Hyattsville, MD: National Center for Health Statistics.

Anderson, G. (2002). *Testimony Before the Subcommittee on Health of the House Committee on Ways and Means. Hearing on Promoting Disease Management in Medicare: 2002* [Online]. http://waysandmeans.house.gov/health

*Administration of Aging.* (2004). *A Profile of Older Americans*. Washington, DC: United States Department of Health and Human Services.

Bales, CW, Buhr, G. (2008). Is Obesity Bad for Older Persons? A Systematic Review of the Pros and Cons of Weight Reduction in Later Life. *Journal of American Medical Association*. 9(5);302—312.

Bartali, B, Frongillo, EA, Bandinelli, S, et al. (2006). Low Nutrient Intake Is an Essential Component of Frailty in Older Persons. *Journals of Gerontology. Series A: Biological Sciences and Medical Sciences*. 61(6);589—593.

Blaum, CS, Xue, QL, Michelon, E, et al. (2005). The Association Between Obesity and the Frailty Syndrome in Older Women: The Women's Health and Aging Studies. *Journal of American Geriatric Society*. 53;927—934.

Cohen, RA, Poppas, A, Forman, DE, et al. (2009). Vascular and Cognitive Functions Associated with Cardiovascular Disease in the Elderly. *Journal of Clinical and Experimental Neuropsychology*. 31(1);96–110.

Colby, SL, Ortman, JM. (2014). *Projections of the Size and Composition of the U.S. Population: 2014 to 2060, Current Population Reports*. U.S. Census Bureau. Washington, DC, P25–1143.

Council on Scientific Affairs. (1990). American Medical Association White Paper on Elderly Health. Report of the Council on Scientific Affairs. *Archives of Internal Medicine*. 150;2459–2472.

Dedeyne, L, Deschodt, M, Verschueren, S, Tournoy, J, Gielen, E. (2017). Effects of Multi-Domain Interventions in (Pre)Frail Elderly on Frailty, Functional, and Cognitive Status: A Systematic Review. *Clinical Interventions in Aging*. 12;873–896.

de Labra, C, Guimaraes-Pinheiro, C, Maseda, A, Lorenzo, T, Millan-Calenti, JC. (2015). Effects of Physical Exercise Interventions in Frail Older Adults: A Systematic Review of Randomized Controlled Trials. *BMC Geriatrics*. 15(154);1–16.

Dey, DK, Lissner, L. (2003). Obesity in 70-Year-Old Subjects as a Risk Factor for 15-Year Coronary Heart Disease Incidence. *Obesity Research*. 11(7);817–827.

Dominguez, LJ, Barbagallo, M. (2017). The Relevance of Nutrition for the Concept of Cognitive Frailty. *Current Opinion in Clinical Nutrition and Metabolic Care*. 20(1);61–68.

Dyeson, TB, Murphy, J, Stryker, K. (1999). Demographic and Psychosocial Characteristics of Cognitively-Intact Chronically Elders Receiving Home Health Services. *Home Health Care Services Quarterly*. 18(2),1–25.

Ershler, WB. (2007). A Gripping Reality: Oxidative Stress, Inflammation, and the Pathway to Frailty. *Journal of Applied Physiology*. 103(1);3–5.

Experton, B, Ozminkowski, RJ, Branch, LG. (1996). A Comparison by Payor/Provider Type of the Cost of Dying Among frail Older Adults. *Journal of American Geriatric Society*. 44(9);1098–1107.

Fairfield, KM, Fletcher, RH. (2002). Vitamins for Chronic Disease Prevention in Adults: Scientific Review. *Journal of American Medical Association*. 287(23);3116–3126.

Fairhall, N, Langron, C, Sherrington, C, et al. (2011). Treating Frailty: A Practical Guide. *BMC Medicine*. 9;83.

Franceschi, C, Garagnani, P, Morsiani, C, Conte, M, Santoro, A, et al. (2018). The Continuum of Aging and Age-Related Diseases: Common Mechanisms but Different Rates. *Frontiers in Medicine*. 5;1–23.

Fried, LP, Ferrucci, L, Darer, J, Williamson, JD, Anderson, G. (2004). Untangling the Concepts of Disability, Frailty, and Comorbidity: Implications for Improved Targeting and Care. *Journal of Gerontology*. 59(3);255–263.

Fried, LP, Guralnik, JM. (1997). Disability in Older Adults: Evidence Regarding Significance, Etiology, and Risk. *Journal of American Geriatric Society*. 45;92–100.

Fried, LP, Kronmal, RA, Newman, AB, et al. (1998). Risk Factors for 5-Year Mortality in Older Adults; The Cardiovascular Health Study. *Journal of American Medical Association*. 279;585–592.

Gabrel, CS. (2000). An Overview of Nursing Home Facilities: Data from the 1997 National Nursing Home Survey. In: *Advance Data from Vital and Health Statistics: No. 311*. Hyattsville, MD: National Center for Health Statistics.

Gates, DM, Succop, P, Brehm, BJ, Gillespie, GL, Sommers, BD. (2008). Obesity and Presenteeism: The Impact of Body Mass Index on Workplace Productivity. *Journal of Occupational and Environmental Medicine*. 50(1);39–45.

Goldman, DP, Cutler, D, Shang, B, Joyce, G. (2005). *The Value of Elderly Disease Prevention*. Washington, DC: Centers for Medicare and Medicaid Services.

Goodpaster, BH, Carlson, CL, Visser, M, Kelley, DE, Scherzinger, A, Harrris, TB, et al. (2001). Attenuation of Skeletal Muscle and Strength in the Elderly: The Health ABC Study. *Journal of Applied Physiology*. 90(6);2157–2165.

Goodpaster, BH, Theriault, R, Watkins, SC, Kelley, DE. (2000). Intramuscular Lipid Content Is Increased in Obesity and Decreased by Weight Loss. *Metabolism*. 49(4);467–472.

Guralnik, JM, Fried, LP, Simonsick, EM, Kasper, JD, Lafferty, ME. (1995). *The Women's Health and Aging Study: Health and Social Characteristics of Older Women with Disability*. Bethesda, MD: National Institute on Aging. NIH Pub, 95–4009.

Guralnik, JM, LaCroix, A, Everett, D, Kovar, M. (1989). *Aging in the Eighties: The Prevalence of Comorbidity and Its Association With Disability. Advance Data From Vital and Health Statistics.* Hyattsville, MD: National Center for Health Statistics.

Guyonnet, S, Secher, M, Vellas, B. (2015). Nutrition, Frailty, Cognitive Frailty and Prevention of Disabilities with Aging. In: Meier, RF, Reddy, BR, Soeters, PB (Editors), *The Importance of Nutrition as an Integral Part of Disease Management, Nestlé Nutrition Institute Workshop.* Basel: Nestec Ltd., Vevey/S. Karger AG. 82;143–152. DOI: 10.1159/000382011

Harris, TB, Launer, LJ, Madans, J, Feldman, JJ. (1997). Cohort Study of Effect of Being Overweight and Change in Weight on Risk of Coronary Heart Disease in Old Age. *British Medical Journal.* 314(7097);1791–1794.

Havighurst, R. (1961). Successful Aging. *Gerontologist.* 1;8–13.

Hoffman, C, Rice, DP. (1996). *Chronic Care in America: A 21st Century Challenge.* San Francisco, CA: The Institute for Health and Aging, University of California.

Hoffman, C, Rice, DP, Sung, HY. (1996). Persons with Chronic Conditions: Their Prevalence and Costs. *Journal of American Medical Association.* 276;1473–1479.

Institute of Medicine. (2008). *Committee on the Future Health Care Workforce for Older Americans. Retooling for an Aging America.* Washington, DC: National Academies Press.

Janssen, I, Shepard, DS, Katzmarzyk, PT, Roubenoff, R. (2004). The Healthcare Costs of Sarcopenia in the United States. *Journal of the American Geriatric Society.* 52;80–85.

Jensen, GL, Hsiao, PY. (2010). Obesity in Older Adults: Relationship to Functional Limitation. *Current Opinion in Clinical Nutrition and Metabolic Care.* 13(1);46–51.

Kelaiditi, E, Cesari, M, Canevelli, M, et al. (2013). Cognitive Frailty: Rational and Definition from an (I.A.N.A./I.A.G.G.) International Consensus Group. *Journal of Nutrition, Health and Aging.* 17(9);726–734.

Khandelwal, D, Goel, A, Kumar, U, et al. (2012). Frailty Is Associated with Longer Hospital Stay and Increased Mortality in Hospitalized Older Patients. *Journal of Nutrition, Health and Aging.* 16;732–735.

Knickman, J, Snell, E. (2002). The 2030 Problem: Caring for the Aging Baby Boomers. *Health Services Research.* 37(4);849–884.

Kobayashi S, Asakura, K, Suga, H, Sasaki, S. (2013). Three-Generation Study of Women on Diets and Health Study Group, High Protein Intake Is Associated With Low Prevalence of Frailty Among Old Japanese Women: A Multicenter Cross-Sectional Study. *Nutrition Journal.* 12;164.

Lane, JS, Magno, CP, Lane, KT, Chan, T, Hoyt, DB, Greenfield, S. (2008). Nutrition Impacts the Prevalence of Peripheral Arterial Disease in the United States. *Journal of Vascular Surgery.* 48(4);897–904.

Merck Institute of Aging and Health, Centers for Disease Control and Prevention. (2004). *The State of Aging and Health in America 2004.* Washington, DC: MIAH.

Mezey, M, Fulmer, T. (1998). Quality Care for the Frail Elderly. *Nursing Outlook.* 46(6);291–292.

Michelon, E, Blaum, C, Semva, RD, Xue, OL, Riks, MO, et al. (2006). Vitamin and Carotenoid Status in Older Women: Associations with the Frailty Syndrome. *Journals of Gerontology. Series A: Biological Sciences and Medical Sciences.* 61(6);600–607.

Moro, C, Galgani, JE, Luu, L, Pasarica, M, Mairal, A, Bajpeyi, S, et al. (2009). Influence of Gender, Obesity, and Muscle Lipase Activity on Intramyocellular Lipids in Sedentary Individuals. *Journal of Clinical Endocrinology and Metabolism.* 94(9);3440–3447.

*National Center for Chronic Disease Prevention and Health Promotion.* (2013). *The State of Aging & Health in America 2013.* Atlanta, GA: Centers for Disease Control and Prevention. US Department of Health and Human Services.

Panza, F, Seripa, D, Solfrizzi, V, et al. (2015). Targeting Cognitive Frailty: Clinical and Neurobiological Roadmap for a Single Complex Phenotype. *Journal of Alzheimer's Disease.* 47(4);793–813.

Pope, A, Tarlov, A. (1991). *Disability in American: Toward a National Agenda for Prevention, Institute of Medicine (U.S.) Committee on a National Agenda for the Prevention of Disabilities.* Washington, DC: National Academies Press.

Puett, D. (2018). Biology of Aging: Identified Drivers and Interventions for Optimal Healthspan. *ACSM's Health & Fitness Journal.* 22;17–27.

Rizzoli, R. (2010). Management of the Oldest Old with Osteoporosis. *European Geriatric Medicine.* 1(1);15–21.

Schmier, JK, Jones, ML, Halpern, MT. (2006). Cost of Obesity in the Workplace. *Scandinavian Journal of Work, Environment & Health.* 32(1);5–11.

Solfrizzi, V, Scafato, E, Frisardi, V, Sancarlo, D, et al. (2012). Frailty Syndrome and All-Cause Mortality in Demented Patients: The Italian Longitudinal Study on Aging. *Age.* 34;507–517.

Starr, KNP, McDonald, SR, Bales, CW. (2014). Obesity and Physical Frailty in Older Adults: A Scoping Review of Intervention Trials. *Journal of the American Medical Directors Association.* 15(4);240–250.

Topinkova, E. (2008). Aging, Disability and Frailty. *Annals of Nutrition and Metabolism.* 52(1);6–11.

*United Nations.* (2015). *World Population Ageing 2015* [Online]. www.un.org/en/development/desa/population/publications/pdf/ageing/WPA2015_Report.pdf

*US Census Bureau. National Population Projections, US Census Web Site* [Online]. www.census.gov/population/www/projections/summarytables.html

Villareal, DT, Banks, M, Sinacore, DR, Siener, C, Klein, S. (2006). Effect of Weight Loss and Exercise on Frailty in Obese Older Adults. *Archives of Internal Medicine.* 166(8);860–866.

Wan, H, Sengupta, M, Velkoff, VA, DeBarrow, KA. (2005). *65+ in the United States: 2005 Current Population Report, P23–209, Washington, DC: US Census Bureau* [Online]. www.census/gov/prod/2006pubs/p23–209.pdf

Woods, AJ, Cohen, RA, Pahor, M. (2013). Cognitive Frailty: Frontiers and Challenges. *Journal of Nutrition, Health and Aging.* 17(9);741–743.

# 3

# PERSPECTIVES FOR HEALTHY AGING AND FRAILTY

The phenotype of frailty (Latin: fragilita; brittleness) refers to an individual's physical appearance (such as sarcopenia, anorexia, and osteoporosis) and physical capacity (i.e., fatigue, risk of falls, and poor health) as a consequence of a decrease in several physiological systems (Clegg & Young 2011). The decrease in functional reserve in frail older individuals is the result of specific homeostatic changes that interact cumulatively and detrimentally following certain stressor events (Strandberg & Pitkala 2007). The vulnerability to sudden changes in health and well-being is determined by the individual's genotype, which is a set of genes adversely influenced by events triggered by environmental stressors.

The sudden and unpredictable change in the health of older frail adults is driven by the interaction of numerous factors that represent a self-perpetuating cycle of structural and physiological events. For example, a low consumption of protein in the diet coupled with physical inactivity can lead to a loss of muscle mass, strength, power, walking speed, exhaustion, falls, disability, anorexia, and other indicators of frailty (Fried & Walston 2003).

## Healthy Aging

Despite the understanding of what constitutes healthy aging, the majority of middle-aged and older adults throughout the United States and worldwide do not engage in regular exercise. In fact, it is clear that many people, regardless of age, gender, and/or financial status, are not interested in exercising or even talking about the health benefits of even minimum physical activity levels to maintain their health and well-being. What is important to most adults is making money, buying a new car, or going on a vacation.

Thus, the association between the frailty syndrome and the clinical adverse health issues is a common clinical condition that should be avoided by aging adults. The development of a physical disability as a result of frailty is not an outcome that should be taken lightly. A good understanding of the physical, mental, nutritional, pharmacological, and biochemical interventions is imperative with aging.

DOI: 10.4324/9781003119920-4

---

## BOX 3.1   CALL TO ACTION.

A call to action or a CTA by the ASEP leadership is critical to improving the health of aging men and women. If you are having health issues, learn more about how ASEP exercise physiologists are interested in helping you. Yes, you can be strong again. You can increase the size and strength of your muscles. Your skeletal system can once again be strong.

For computer access, take a look at the following URLs:

*ASEP's Exercise Medicine Text for Exercise Physiologists* (benthambooks.com)

Read ASEPs exercise medicine text for exercise physiologists Full Book (book247all.com)

**American Society of Exercise Physiologists** recognize the need for regular exercise. The ASEP organization is 100% committed to the health and well-being of society by developing healthcare professionals as ASEP Board-Certified Exercise Physiologists who will prescribe exercise medicine to (a) boost activity levels, (b) increase muscle strength and flexibility, and (d) elevate mood of aging adults to help them maintain and/or improve their quality of life and avoid unhealthy days of mental depression and/or impairment, muscle and/or joint pain and disability.

---

Aging, frailty, and the effects on the mind and body are not topics of great interest even though exercise improves health, reduces the risk of falls, and improves balance. Yet, ironically, at a time when knowledge of the aging human body with and without regular physical activity is important for health reasons, adults are graduating from high school and/or college and doing whatever they can to enjoy life except engaging in regular exercise. Physical activity is a huge void in their education, work environment, and life at home. Although this is true for all individuals regardless of their age, it is not a healthy way to live.

---

## BOX 3.2   AS A BEGINNING POINT, HOW MUCH ACTIVITY DO ADULTS NEED?

* 150 min of **aerobic** activity every week to keep the heart and lungs healthy. This could be 30 min of walking 5 d·wk$^{-1}$ or 50 min of walking 3 d·wk$^{-1}$.
* 2 or more days of **anaerobic** activity (i.e., resistance training) every week to keep the muscles of the arms, shoulders, chest, abdomen, back, hips, and legs strong.

---

It is common knowledge that the majority of young children, high school and college students, and their parents do not exercise. This fact alone threatens the health and well-being of young men and women growing up in the United States and worldwide. Exercise medicine along with eating fruits and vegetables daily represents a viable and scientifically proven way to reduce the risk of some cancers and chronic diseases, mental depression, and frailty. It is for this reason that improvement in society's thinking regarding health issues is imperative. Here, the point is that it is not a question of developing new drugs and/or surgical procedures to deal with health problems. What is important is that the educational system and the parental oversight of "what it means to be healthy" must highlight the power of regular exercise to keep the human body healthy.

Families should raise their children with an emphasis on how muscles work, how they move, how exercise helps to avoid obesity, and how to reduce the risk factors for many chronic conditions (such as heart disease, stroke, arthritis, and disabilities). Having such knowledge at a young age and throughout adulthood will help everyone to better understand the importance of exercise medicine.

Hence, while clinics and hospital-centered medical treatments are important for obvious reasons, adults in particular should take the initiative to avoid the leading causes of illness and death by living a healthier lifestyle. They can do this by accessing a qualified teacher with a healthcare-oriented education and experience with what constitutes a safe exercise program.

Because walking is the most common type of exercise to maintain a certain level of personal health-related quality of life, it is important that public health strategies in age-friendly communities contribute to increased opportunities to walk safely and independently to help decrease obesity and increase healthy aging of older adults (Hoehner et al. 2005; Wilcox et al. 2000). Such programs will also help older adults age well with minimal or no limitations in mobility (impaired mobility), thus decreasing the risk of depression, falls, and the risk of death.

It should be obvious, but it isn't always the case. Adults who are aging in a healthy way are not frail. They are optimistic, eat healthy foods, and have a spring in their step. Non-frail adults, which represents ~90% of Americans aged 65 and older, have a lower risk of infections, illnesses that are treated in the hospital, and falls. They experience less risk of surgical complications and days in the hospital as well as a decrease in the odds of living in a nursing home or assisted living facility.

Healthy aging is essentially the opposite of frailty. Thus, the bodyweight of non-frail adults looks good for their height. They do not look like they are shrinking, and they have not lost 10 or more pounds in the past year. Aging without frailty does not automatically render adults weak. That is, they do not need help to stand up, and if they wish to pick up a package and/or engage in household chores they have the grip strength to do so as well.

## Aging, Physical Activity, and Health

The National Population Projections Report indicates that the year 2030 will mark a demographic turning point in which all baby boomers will be older than 65 years. This means that one in every five adult residents will be retirement age. By 2035, there will be 78 million people 65 years and older compared to 76.7 million under the age of 18 (U.S. Census Bureau 2018).

These unprecedented demographic transitions are very important. In fact, they are critically important, given the challenges of limited healthcare resources and the insufficient attention regarding quality of life, the frailty syndrome, and the fact that more than one in four Americans are living with multiple, concurrent, chronic conditions (U.S. Department of Health and Human Services 2010).

As an ASEP exercise physiologist, the question is "What are the ASEP innovative approaches to caring for the health and well-being of persons aged 65 years and older?" Without question, the aging of the population will have wide-ranging healthcare implications. The projected growth of the older population in the United States will present challenges to Social Security and Medicare as well as have a major influence on families and businesses. ASEP exercise physiologists are poised to help promote successful aging of adults by assisting in the development of community-based safe walking programs and fitness-based programs to maintain or improve the aging adults' cognitive behavioral health, physical functioning, mobility, and balance.

---

**BOX 3.3    AS THE NUMBER OF AGING ADULTS INCREASES, ASEP EXERCISE PHYSIOLOGISTS WILL. . .**

- Find innovative ways to deal with the different needs of the aging adult population;
- Identify timely steps and procedures by which the profession of exercise physiology will address the healthcare opportunities created by the aging U.S. population;
- Identify and explain how to avoid a higher body mass index due to fatness and weaker thigh muscles associated with aging;
- Educate older adults on the "psychophysiology" of exercise medicine, particularly the significance of increased cardiorespiratory and metabolic function; and
- Focus on the education of "Healthy Aging" to improve the health and functioning of older adults so they will be able to lead a healthy life relatively free from illness or disability.

ASEP Board-Certified Exercise Physiologists are essential healthcare professionals. This point is emphasized in hundreds of articles published in the ASEP electronic journal, the ***Professionalization of Exercise Physiologists-online***(URL: American Society of Exercise Physiologists—Professionalization of Exercise Physiology (asep.org)).

---

It was previously thought in 2012 that data from the UK Office for National Statistics indicated the number of people who were over 85 years of age would increase from 1.4 million to around 3.5 million by 2035 (McPhee et al. 2016). Regardless of the inter-individual variability in health and the onset of muscular weakness, disability, and frailty, aging is increasingly associated with a progressive decline in cognitive function and numerous other age-related declines in the structure and function of cardiorespiratory, metabolic, and skeletal muscle systems. The effect is frequently an unintentional weight loss, a low level of physical activity, decreased gait speed, exhaustion, and weakness.

The future of aging can continue with increased frailty and individuals with reduced mental and physical function or it can be one of living longer with good health due to the adaptations of the physiological systems to regular exercise. Society has a choice. Middle-aged adults can grow older while taking responsibility for their health, which will result in a healthy cardiorespiratory system to more effectively distribute oxygen to all parts of the body. Or, once again, they can continue to turn a blind eye to the health benefits of exercise medicine.

---

**BOX 3.4    WHAT DOES RESEARCH SAY ABOUT A LOW LEVEL OF PHYSICAL ACTIVITY?**

- In **2008,** Nazroo et al. reported that sedentary adults 50 years of age and older had twice the risk of death when compared to other adults in the same age group who were physically active.

- In **2011**, the Department of Culture carried out a survey of >92,000 people in England. The findings showed that participation in exercise decreased progressively during adult life. The decrease was influenced by the lack of desire to engage in physical activity.
- In **2012**, Lee et al. reported that physical inactivity was the primary cause of poor fitness in older adults, and that the effect of inactivity was equal to the effects of smoking, obesity, and excessive intake of alcohol.
- In **2014**, Matthews et al. reported that adults who retired from work were more likely to change to low levels of physical exercise from high and medium levels than those who remained in work.

Contrary to the findings in Box 3.4, adults with a lower risk of mortality had a higher cardiorespiratory fitness level due to their high level of physical activity. In other words, better health (Hamer et al. 2014) and longevity (Manini et al. 2006) are logical outcomes of maintaining a physically active lifestyle that decreases cholesterol, blood pressure, and the risk of cardiovascular and metabolic disease (Earnest et al. 2013).

Cognitive function is also a primary area of benefit from regular exercise along with an improvement in balance and coordination that helps to decrease the risk of falls and disabilities (Franco et al. 2014; Gillespie et al. 2012; Lautenschlager et al. 2008). In particular, regular resistance training strengthens the skeletal system by increasing bone mineral density (Ireland et al. 2014), which helps to decrease the chance of fractures. The evidence is clear. All older adults, especially those with frailty, need to be more physically active.

The intensity of exercise does not have to be vigorous to help reduce the risk of developing frailty or chronic diseases. Low-to-moderate-intensity aerobic exercise (such as walking 150 min·wk$^{-1}$) is low risk for most adults and sufficient to decrease the risk of morbidity, mortality, and functional dependence (Chou et al. 2014). In fact, Ferrucci et al. (1999) reported that walking 5 to 7 d·wk$^{-1}$ increased longevity by ~4 years and disability-free life expectancy by ~2 years. It is also important that older adults engage in low-to-moderate-intensity resistance training to increase the size and strength of the muscles of the upper and lower limbs to protect against the effects of sarcopenia. The loss of lean muscle mass, strength, and endurance with aging predisposes adults of all ages, especially older adults to daily mobility issues (Harridge et al. 1999).

Combining walking and strengthening exercises is better than just walking or just lifting weights. Doing both anaerobic and aerobic exercises not only builds strength and aerobic endurance throughout the musculoskeletal and cardiorespiratory systems, respectively. The overall effect of doing both significantly improves quality of life more so than walking alone (Pahor et al. 2014).

## Social and Treatment Implications

With all the scientific information about aging, frailty, and the importance of regular exercise, why would middle-aged and older adults continue to live a sedentary lifestyle with the obvious health expectations of doing so? The answer may be found in the Department of Health Report that says exercise habits differ depending on the adults' age, gender, ethnicity, income, and disability. The Report states that a high level of physical activity is more likely to be valued and maintained by older adults of a high socioeconomic position (Department of Health

2011). In support of the Report, Matthews et al. (2014) indicated that older adults of a low socioeconomic position are less interested in exercising. Also, it is interesting that Hamer et al. (2014) reported that adults from more affluent backgrounds were almost three times more likely to be healthy in older age than adults from less affluent backgrounds. Without question, there is a relationship between the health of older adults and socioeconomic position.

McPhee et al. (2016) reported in *Biogerontology* that Sport-England (2006) had concluded the motivation for sports participation consisted of internal reasons (such as personal health, mental and emotional benefits, and social) and external reasons (such as friends and/or family, partners, doctors, and the media). Sports-England (2006) also stated the cultural norms, language barriers, costs, safety, and whether the exercise is enjoyable and safe as factors that predicted initiation and maintenance of an exercise program. No doubt there are many reasons for not starting an exercise program. French (2013) and van Stralen et al. (2010) indicated that self-efficacy (i.e., belief in one's ability to start and carry out an exercise program) is important in the initiation of an exercise program and whether the program will produce positive results, respectively.

There are other factors as well that influence whether an older adult will be part of an exercise program. For example, is the purpose of the exercise program to have fun or is it for health reasons (Devereux-Fitzgerald et al. 2016)? Is it a walking program (Kassavou et al. 2013) or is it a sports-oriented exercise program (Hunt et al. 2014)? Is there the opportunity to interact socially with other adults (Koeneman et al. 2011), and how much does it cost to be part of the program (Sallis & Owen 1998)? Regardless of the motivating reason to participate in an exercise program, McPhee et al. (2016) conclude that older adults may be encouraged to engage in an exercise medicine program if the cost is low, has a fun element to it, and if they are told to do so by a medical professional.

Regardless of the different factors and feelings about this or that, the research data point to the obvious fact. That is, to slow the aging rate, it is imperative that middle-aged and older adults adopt a lifestyle that helps them to stay healthy and active as long as possible. Exercise medicine is the answer to living longer and healthier. It not only strengthens the mind and body to deal with stressors but also reduces the inevitable suffering, disabilities, and dependence that are linked to aging. Thus, for every person regardless of age, sex, and/or country, to live a healthier and longer life than expected, it is the responsibility of every adult to engage in regular exercise to minimize the progressive accumulation of molecular damage associated with aging. After all, it is increasingly becoming clear that we are a nation of adults who were 1 in every 25 Americans in 1900 to 1 in 8 in 1994. Twenty-five years later, it is anticipated that the elderly population will more than double between 2019 and the year 2050 to 80 million (i.e., 1 in 5 Americans will be elderly). Simply put the increase in older adults will continue to highlight the geriatric syndrome of increased vulnerability to chronic diseases and disabilities.

Regular exercise can help maintain a healthy body composition, homoeostatic regulation, and energetic power. The appropriate prescription of exercise medicine can help prevent accelerated aging, decrease the likelihood of psychosocial and medical adverse outcomes, dependency, and the necessity for institutional stay and hospitalizations. It is crucial that healthcare professionals anticipate the increase in the functional challenges faced by older adults, and especially that we appreciate Americans are reaching increasingly advanced ages. The segment of the population of individuals aged 90 years and older is not only the fastest growing in the United States, but He and Muenchrath (2011) reported that this age range is expected to quadruple in size from 2010 to 2050 and will comprise a greater proportion of the U.S. total population than ever before.

---

**BOX 3.5 THE ASEP HEALTHCARE TREATMENT FOR FRAILTY PATIENTS.**

When diagnosed with frailty, it is important that an ASEP Board-Certified Exercise Physiologist is available in existing geriatric centers as part of the healthcare team's approach to helping correct frailty in the elderly. While it is not too common to have exercise physiologists on the healthcare team, it is imperative that they are part of the team. Frailty can be prevented or treated with exercise, diet, and good medical care. The exercise physiologist is educated and certified to work as part of the healthcare team to improve the frail person's health status.

---

## Demographic Trends, Aging, and Concerns

As indicated in earlier sections, the age structure of the U.S. population is expected to change over the coming decades. In 2050, the population aged 65 and over is projected to be 83.7 million, which is almost double its estimated population of 43.1 million in 2012 (Ortman et al. 2014). Not only will the graying of American become more racially and ethnically diverse but also the cost and quality of the geriatric care will be an important healthcare concern. By 2030, more than 20% of U.S. residents are projected to be 65 years of age and over, compared to 13% in 2010 and 9.8% in 1970.

Two important reasons (e.g., public health campaigns and behavioral changes) for the increase in percent of projected adults 65 years of age and over are the drivers of decreased mortality: smoking and obesity. For example, the American Lung Association (2011) reported that in 1970 45% of the U.S. population between 25 and 44 years of age smoked. This age range represents adults who are between 67 and 86 years of age in 2012. In 2011, 22.1% of the adults aged 25 to 44 smoked, which will be the population aged 64 to 83 in 2050 (Centers for Disease Control and Prevention 2012). The bottom line is very important: the decrease in younger individuals' smoking is expected to improve their survivorship when they reach the older age range.

It is a deeply felt joy to know that the future will encompass older individuals who either never smoked or stopped early due to concerns about health. It is noteworthy that these aging adults will still be vulnerable to everyday stressors. They and the various medical interventions will still be a critical part of their means of dealing with disease and/or disability. In fact, many aging adults will still be subject to complex and equivocal treatment.

Understandably, there is no absolute 1, 2, 3 this or that to avoid health problems. What we do know is this: A healthy transition into the older years is better than aging with little to no attention given to the risk factors that drive certain mental and physical diseases and/or disabilities. Clearly, all adults should be responsible for recognizing an unhealthy lifestyle. Otherwise the inevitable is statistically just around the corner which most frail elderly adults can expect to experience (i.e., delirium, falls, immobility, and incontinence) (Jarrett et al. 1995). Of interest is the fact that these four outcomes are linked to the poor control and/or integration of a higher order of cognitive processing that allows for standing upright, maintaining balance, and walking without falling (Rockwood 1997).

Without question, the inability to walk short distances is an important clue to the mental and physical status of the frail elderly people. There are also other clues, such as complex alterations of pharmacokinetics and pharmacodynamics along with a reduced physiologic reserve that decreases the aging adult's ability to compensate for disruptions to hemostasis. Hence, the abnormal frail adult's interplay of genetics, biological, and environmental factors contribute to higher levels of frailty that is associated with an increased risk of death.

The connection between chronic, low-level inflammation and age-related hormonal and metabolic alterations is considered to be key pathogenic factor in physical frailty's coexistent with cognitive frailty and cognitive impairment (Soysal et al. 2016; Fougere et al. 2017). Also, it is believed that women may be more prone to higher inflammatory markers than men (Gordon & Hubbard 2018), and they may experience more chronic, low-level inflammation and frailty than men because they have more abdominal fat in older age (Hubbard et al. 2010; Stevens et al. 2010).

The sedentary lifestyle, aging, and frailty represent a problem in society that is not going away, especially since the world population is projected to reach 9.9 billion by 2050, that is, a 29% increase (2.3 billion people) from an estimated 7.6 billion now (Kaneda et al. 2018). Similarly, Kaneda et al. (2018) indicate that the Population Reference Bureau (PRB) projects that Africa's population will more than double to 2.6 billion by 2050. Asia is expected to increase by 717 million to 5.3 billion. Also, the PRB projects that by 2050, 16% of the world population will be 65 and older (a 9% increase).

---

### BOX 3.6   KANEDA ET AL. (2018) INDICATE THAT THE AGE DATA AND ANALYSIS SHOW:

- Eighty-two countries are projected by 2050 to have at least 20% of their population ages ≥65, which is an increase of 13 countries in 32 years.
- By 2050, the Northern Africa population of 65 and older is projected to nearly quadruple.
- The percentage of the population age ≥65 in the United States is projected to increase from 15% in 2018 to 22% in 2050.
- In Japan, more than 36% of the population is projected to be ≥65 years of age by 2050.

---

## Final Thoughts

Since diverse psychological and social factors appear to contribute to certain social and cognitive issues with aging, it is imperative that older adults are educated to deal with the medical syndrome. In particular, elderly people should recognize their responsibility to integrate a cognitive intervention and nutritional supplementation approach with a strong commitment to regular aerobic exercise (at 70% of maximum heart rate) and moderate-intensity resistance training (5 to 6 on a 0 to 10 scale) to avoid a sedentary lifestyle and reduce falls.

As with any medication, the effectiveness of exercise medicine is subject to the right intensity prescription and adherence. Ultimately, there will be improvement in walking status and functional activity of frail older adults by improving aerobic capacity, muscle mass, strength, and gait speed to help them live longer without hospitalization, nursing home placement, and a high cost of physical and/or mental (psychological care).

Frailty affects ~20% of all older adults (Robinson et al. 2015). With the population aged ≥60 growing faster than all the younger age groups, frailty will increasingly become a major clinical condition with significant adverse health outcomes. The contribution of physiological, muscular, cognitive, and nutritional support from ASEP Board-Certified Exercise Physiologists in the prevention of falls and delirium in older age with the exercise medicine intervention will be critical to their well-being. In fact, given the multiple morbidities, functional, and psychological impairments within the aging populations, professional support services will be a major concern.

Looking to the 21st century regarding aging, the United Nations (2017) indicates that the aging of the population is one of the most challenging social issues the world will confront. The Aging Report states there are an estimated 962 million people 60 years of age or older in the world in 2017, which makes up 13% of the global population. Without question, rapid aging is occurring throughout the world. The Report indicates that the number of older persons in the world is projected to be 1.4 billion in 2030 and 2.1 billion in 2050, and could rise to 3.1 billion in 2100. Also, globally, the number of persons 80 years of age or older is expected to triple by 2050 (i.e., from 137 million in 2017 to 425 million in 2050). By 2100, it is expected to increase to 909 million, which is ~7 times its value in 2017.

The essential feature of health care to meet the needs of increasingly frail aging adults is a seamless interface between the academic institutions and healthcare professionals. The quality of care can be significantly improved with the guidance and supervision of ASEP Board-Certified Exercise Physiologists. In fact, the future of long-term care of acceptable quality likely depends on a mixture of exercise medicine by exercise physiologists and geriatricians who also have a vital role in tailoring services to individual needs.

## References

*American Lung Association.* (2011). *Trends in Tobacco Use.* Chicago, IL: American Lung Association, Research and Program Services, Epidemiology and Statistics Unit.

*American Society of Exercise Physiologists.* (2016). Professionalization of Exercise Physiology-Online [Online]. www.asep.org/resources/pep-online/

*Centers for Disease Control and Prevention.* (2012). Current Cigarette Smoking Among Adults. United States, 2011, Morbidity and Mortality Weekly Report. 61(44);889–894.

Chou, WT, Tomata, Y, Watanabe, T, et al. (2014). Relationships Between Changes in Time Spent Walking Since Middle Age and Incident Functional Disability. *Preventive Medicine.* 59;68–72.

Clegg, A, Young, J. (2011). The Frailty Syndrome. *Clinical Medicine.* 11(1);72–75.

*Department of Health UK.* (2011). *Start Active, Stay Active: UK Physical Activity Guidelines* [Online]. www.dh.gov.uk/health/category/publications/

Devereux-Fitzgerald, A, Powell, R, Dewhurst, A, French, D. (2016). The Acceptability of Physical Activity Interventions to Older Adults: A Systematic Review and Meta-Synthesis. *Social Science Medicine.* 158;14–23.

Earnest, CP, Johannsen, NM, Swift, DL, et al. (2013). Dose Effect of Cardiorespiratory Exercise on Metabolic Syndrome in Postmenopausal Women. *American Journal of Cardiology.* 111;1805–1811.

Ferrucci, L, Izmirlian, G, Leveille, S, et al. (1999). Smoking, Physical Activity, and Active Life Expectancy. *American Journal of Epidemiology.* 149;645–653.

Fougere, B, Boulanger, E, Nourthashemi, F, et al. (2017). Chronic Inflammation: Accelerator of Biological Aging. *Journal of Gerontology: Series A Biological Sciences and Medical Sciences.* 72(9);1218–1225.

Franco, MR, Pereira, LS, Ferreira, PH. (2014). Exercise Interventions for Preventing Falls in Older People Living in the Community. *British Journal of Sports Medicine.* 48;867–868.

French, DP. (2013). The Role of Self-Efficacy in Changing Health-Related Behavior: Cause, Effect or Spurious Association? *British Journal of Health Psychology.* 18;237–243.

Fried, L, Walston, J. (2003). Frailty and Failure to Thrive. In: Hazzard, W, Blass, J, Halter, J, et al. (Editors), *Principles of Geriatric Medicine and Gerontology* (5th Edition). New York, NY: McGraw-Hill.

Gillespie, LD, Robertson, MC, Gillespie, WJ, et al. (2012). Interventions for Preventing Falls in Older People Living in the Community. *Cochrane Database Systematic Review.* 9;CD007146.

Gordon, EH, Hubbard, RE. (2018). Physiological Basis for Sex Differences in Frailty. *Current Opinion in Physiology.* 6;10–15.

Hamer, M, Lavoie, KL, Bacon, SL. (2014). Taking Up Physical Activity in Later Life and Healthy Ageing: The English Longitudinal Study of Ageing. *British Journal of Sports Medicine.* 48;239–243.

Harridge, SD, Kryger, A, Stensgaard, A. (1999). Knee Extensor Strength, Activation, and Size in Very Elderly People Following Strength Training. *Muscle Nerve.* 22;831–839.

He, W, Muenchrath, MN. (2011). 90+ in the United States: 2006–2008. *US Census* [Online]. www.census.gov/library/publications/2011/acs/acs-17.html

Hoehner, CM, Brennan Ramirex, LK, Elliott, MB, et al. (2005). Perceived and Objective Environmental Measures and Physical Activity Among Urban Adults. *American Journal of Preventive Medicine.* 28;105–116.

Hubbard, R, Lang, I, Liewellyn, D, et al. (2010). Frailty, Body Mass Index, and Abdominal Obesity in Older People. *Journal of Gerontology A Biological Sciences and Medical Sciences.* 65(4);377–381.

Hunt, K, Wyke, S, Gray, CM, et al. (2014). A Gender-Sensitized Weight Loss and Healthy Living Program for Overweight and Obese Men Delivered by Scottish Premier League Football Clubs (FFIT): A Pragmatic Randomized Controlled Trial. *Lancet.* 383;1211–1221.

Ireland, A, Maden-Wilkinson, T, Ganse, B, et al. (2014). Effects of Age and Starting Age Upon Side Asymmetry in the Arms of Veteran Tennis Players: A Cross-Sectional Study. *Osteoporosis International.* 25;1389–1400.

Jarrett, PG, Rockwood, K, Carver, D, Stolee, P, Cosway, S. (1995). Illness Presentation in Elderly Patients. *Canadian Medical Association.* 150;489–495.

Kaneda, T, Greenbaum, C, Patierno, K. (2018). PRB Projects 2.3 Billion More People Living on Earth by 2050. *Population Reference Bureau* [Online]. www.prb.org/2018-world-population-data-sheet-with-focus-on-changing-age-structures/

Kassavou, A, Turner, A, French, DP. (2013). Do Interventions to Promote Walking in Groups Increase Physical Activity? A Meta-Analysis. *International Journal of Behavior and Physical Activity.* 10.

Koeneman, MA, Verheijden, MW, Chinapaw, MJ, et al. (2011). Determinants of Physical Activity and Exercise in Healthy Older Adults: A Systematic Review. *International Journal of Behavioral Nutrition and Physical Activity.* 8;142.

Lautenschlager, NT, Cox, KL, Flicker, L, et al. (2008). Effect of Physical Activity on Cognitive Function in Older Adults at Risk for Alzheimer Disease: A Randomized Trial. *Journal of American Medical Association.* 300;1027–1037.

Lee, IM, Shiroma, EJ, Lobelo, F, Puska, P, Blair, SN, Katzmarzyk, PT. (2012). Effect of Physical Inactivity on Major Non-Communicable Diseases Worldwide: An Analysis of Burden of Disease and Life Expectancy. *Lancet.* 380;219–229.

Manini, TM, Everhart, JE, Patel, KV, et al. (2006). Daily Activity Energy Expenditure and Mortality Among Older Adults. *Journal of American Medical Association.* 296;171–179.

Matthews, K, Demakakos, P, Nazroo, J, Shankar, A. (2014). The Evolution of Lifestyles in Older Age in England. In: Banks, J, Nazroo, J, Steptoe, A (Editors), *The Dynamics of Ageing: Evidence From the English Longitudinal Study of Ageing 2002–2012.* London: The Institute for Fiscal Studies, ISBN, 978-1-909463-58-5, 51–93.

McPhee, JS, French, DP, Jackson, D, et al. (2016). Physical Activity in Older Age: Perspectives for Healthy Ageing and Frailty. *Biogerontology.* 17;567–580.

Nazroo, J, Zaninotto, P, Gjonca, E. (2008). Mortality and Healthy Life Expectancy. In: Banks, J, Breeze, E, Lessof, C, Nazroo, J (Editors), *Living in the 21st Century: Older People in England, The 2006 English Longitudinal Study of Ageing.* London: The Institute for Fiscal Studies, 253–288.

Ortman, JM, Velkoff, VA, Hogan, H. (2014). An Aging Nation: The Older Population in the United States: Population Estimates and Projections. *U.S. Census Bureau.* 1–28 [Online]. https://www.census.gov/prod/2014pubs/p25-1140.pdf

Pahor, M, Guralnik, JM, Ambrosius, WT, et al. (2014). Effect of Structured Physical Activity on Prevention of Major Mobility Disability in Older Adults: The LIFE Study Randomized Clinical Trial. *Journal of American Medical Association*. 31;2387–2396.

Robinson, TN, Walston, JD, Brummel, NE, et al. (2015). Frailty for Surgeons: Review of a National Institute on Aging Conference on Frailty for Specialists. *Journal of American College of Surgeons*. 221(6);1083–1092.

Rockwood, K. (1997). Medical Management of Frailty: Confessions of a Gnostic. *Canadian Medical Association*. 157;1081–1084.

Sallis, J, Owen, N. (1998). *Physical Activity and Behavioral Medicine*. Thousand Oaks: Sage.

Soysal, P, Stubbs, B, Lucato, P, et al. (2016). Inflammation and Frailty in the Elderly: A Systematic Review and Meta-Analysis. *Ageing Research Reviews*. 31;1–8.

Sport-England. (2006). *Understanding Participation in Sport: What Determines Sports Participation Among Recently Retired People?* [Online]. www.sportengland.org/medial/39497/understand ing-participation-among-recently-retired-people.pdf

Stevens, J, Katz, E, Huxley, R. (2010). Associations Between Gender, Age, and Waist Circumference. *European Journal of Clinical Nutrition*. 64;6–15.

Strandberg, TE, Pitkala, KH. (2007). Frailty in Elderly People. *Lancet*. 369;1328–1329.

United Nations. (2017). *Ageing* [Online]. www.un.org/en/sections/issues-depth/ageing/

US Census Bureau. (2018). *Older People Expected to Outnumber Children for the First Time in U.S. History* [Online]. www.census.gov/newsroom/press-releases/2018/cb18-41-popula tion-projections.html

US Department of Health and Human Services. (2010). *Multiple Chronic Conditions: A Strategic Framework, Optimum Health and Quality of Life for Individuals with Multiple Chronic Conditions*. Washington, DC: US Department of Health and Human Services [Online]. www.hhs. gov/ash/Initiatives/mcc/mcc_ framework.pdf

Van Stralen, MM, Lechner, L, Mudde, AN, et al. (2010). Determinants of Awareness, Initiation and Maintenance of Physical Activity Among the Over-Fifties: A Delphi Study. *Health Education Research*. 25;233–247.

Wilcox, S, Castro, C, King, AC, et al. (2000). Determinants of Leisure Time Physical Activity in Rural Older and Ethnically Diverse Women in the United States. *Journal of Epidemiology and Community Health*. 54;667–672.

# PART II

# Challenges of Caring for the Frail Elderly

# 4

# THE AGING OF THE BABY BOOMERS

The number of adults born between 1946 and 1964 (the baby boom) is anticipated to have a major impact on the long-term service and support provided by family members. The expectation is that the support of family caregivers is not going to keep up with the future needs of the baby boom. Redfoot et al. (2013) highlight this point in the AARP Public Policy Institute publication in which they state that the number of individuals between 45 and 64 (the primary caregiving years) is expected to decrease (Box 4.1). Yet the overall healthcare needs of adults aged 80 and older will increase. The decline in the availability of family members, partners, and close friends as caregivers will be the primary reason older adults will not be able to stay in their own home when they become frail and disabled. This is just one problem. Aging of adults needs a public health response.

---

**BOX 4.1 LONG-TERM SERVICES WILL NOT MEET THE NEEDS OF OLDER FRAIL ADULTS.**

By 2030, the support of caregivers aged 45 to 64 is expected to decrease to 4 to 1 for each person aged 80 and older, and is expected to decrease to less than 3 to 1 in 2050 when all boomers will be in the high-risk years of life.

—Redfoot, D, Feinberg, L, Houser, A. (2013). The Aging of the Baby Boom and the Growing Care Gap: A Look at Future Declines in the Availability of Family Caregivers. *AARP Public Policy Institute.* 85;1–12.

---

As a result of the decrease in family support in maintaining independence, more frail adults 80 years of age and older will spend more money on assistance for caregivers. The increase in age, frailty, disability, and the need for assistance are all linked to requiring help when getting dressed, preparing meals, going to the bathroom, using the phone and/or computer, and

DOI: 10.4324/9781003119920-6

paying bills (Bault 2012). Being married helps the baby boom because the spouse and grown children often provide the care and support.

All is good except for the time elapse between 2010 and 2030 when the caregivers grow older and become the 80+ population. This means that the actual number of caregivers will decrease (Faureault & Smith 2004), which begs the question: Who is going to take care of the 18 million 80-year-olds in 2030 with the likelihood of disability? In 2010, the 80+ population was 11 million. The increase of 7 million 80-year-olds in 2030 is a concern that continues to increase because the 80+ population is expected to increase by 44% between 2030 and 2040 (Redfoot et al. 2013), while the caregivers aged 45 to 65 is expected to increase only by 10%. This is a critical decrease in assistance to people aged 80 and older.

---

**BOX 4.2   THE CAREGIVERS NOW AND IN THE FUTURE.**

"From 7 potential caregivers per frail older person today . . . to just 4 in 2030 . . . to widen even more as the ratio continues declining to 2.9 by 2050, when we have three times as many people aged 80 and older as there are today."

—Redfoot, D, Feinberg, L, Houser, A. (2013). The Aging of the Baby Boom and The Growing Care Gap: A Look at Future Declines in the Availability of Family Caregivers, *AARP Public Policy Institute.* 85;1–12.

---

## The Future and Senior Care

Aging of the population is both a success story and a worldwide health problem. The challenges created by the aging populations from around the world are real. They not only have a direct impact on the elderly frail person's quality of life but also place a heavy burden of care on the Baby Boomers. Hence, in the anticipation of the future, the period of "old age" is going to be much different from what we know today (Cook 2012).

Developing the skills and being prepared to assume the caregiving role is not easy. It is more often than not a constant uphill challenge that can have a negative influence on the emotional, physical, and financial aspects of the caregiver. From providing unpaid care for the frail older adults to experiencing extreme stress, symptoms of depression, and premature aging, providing care to meet the needs of the aging Baby Boomers is hard and stressful work. Interestingly, the ASEP Board-Certified Exercise Physiologists are in an excellent position to become recognized along with physicians, nurses, and allied healthcare professionals in addressing the needs of the older frail population.

Exercise physiologists are in an excellent position to help in preventing frailty as well as helping the elderly frail adult through difficult physical difficulties by empowering, guiding, teaching, and supporting clients and/or patients as they adapt to an exercise medicine program. In time, with better integration of healthcare collaborations and services by physicians and exercise physiology professionals, more families will be prepared to remain in their homes as they age. The ASEP Board-Certified Exercise Physiologists will help the seniors and frail adults by providing the care that they need, which is cost-effective health and fitness support services to improve their lifestyles.

As a result of the expected increase in health, fitness, and well-being, the boomers will be in a better position to shower, dress, and move about their home and yard without falling and possibly suffering a fracture. Exercise physiologists will not only add to the caregiver supply but also be part of the 21st-century healthcare industry that is specialized in dealing with the mind and body to keep frail adults out of the emergency room, assisted living facilities, residential communities, and nursing homes. This point is extremely important since about 13% of the population (i.e., 42 million seniors) is living today in America, and it is growing at a rapid rate. By 2030, seniors are expected to increase to ~20% of the population, which is again the reason for more and better senior caregivers to avoid the consequences of aging and frailty.

---

**BOX 4.3  BABY BOOMERS, EXERCISE PHYSIOLOGISTS, AND HEALTH CARE.**

The **ASEP Board-Certified Exercise Physiologists** are specifically trained to evaluate and manage the unique healthcare needs and treatment preferences of older people. If they suspect a problem related to lifestyle, whether it is nutrition- and/or physical-related concerns or mental health issues, the ASEP position is that exercise medicine can help improve the senior's mental status (particularly anxiety and depression that can have a positive influence on cognitive skills), and obviously they can promote physiological improvement the reserve capacity of multiple body systems to prevent a decrease in health and wellness.

---

The boom in seniors is real, and it is problematic for many reasons. But it can be helped by credible healthcare professionals, such as by exercise physiologists who graduate with a degree in exercise physiology from an ASEP accredited academic institution (American Society of Exercise Physiologists 2019a). Their presence will allow the older adults to have the opportunity for a community-based mental support and exercise medicine programs to decrease pain, to improve function, and to decrease the risks of chronic conditions such as diabetes, high cholesterol, and hypertension.

Unfortunately, the current approach for the majority of elders who live beyond 75 and 85 years of age is to become frail at some point without doing anything to make a difference in their health. That is, aside from failing to engage in a regular walking and resistance training program, they end up personally accounting for significant out-of-pocket expenses for long-term care.

---

**BOX 4.4  PROJECTIONS OF NATIONAL LONG-TERM CARE EXPENDITURES FOR THE ELDERLY.**

Estimates by the Congressional Budget Office (CBO) indicate that long-term care expenditures were more than $120 billion in 2000, with ~60% of the expenses covered by the public sector. Private insurance covered 1% of the long-term care costs, which out-of-pocket expenses accounted for essentially all of the balance. CBO indicated that total long-term care expenses will increase at a rate of 2.6% per year about inflation over the next 30 years, to $154 billion in 2010, $195 billion in 2020, and $270 billion in 2030.

—*Congressional Budget Office*. (1999). *CBO Memorandum: Projections of Expenditures for Long-Term Care Services for the Elderly.* Washington, DC.

While it is difficult to construct a counterargument to the financial concerns of long-term care and the shrinking of resources in the future, there is the expectation that today's increased emphasis on exercise medicine will have a positive impact on the financial burden of aging and long-term care. There is also the argument that the Baby Boom generation is healthier than other generations (Knickman & Snell 2002), and that the healthy elderly are likely to work longer.

With more young adults taking responsibility for their health status, there should be a decrease in the disability rate as well as the burden of long-term care as they transition into their elderly years. It is anticipated that many of these adults will seek out the expertise of the ASEP exercise physiologist to keep them healthy and strong to decrease the risk of becoming frail or socially isolated. This decision will help keep the financial burden of long-term care moderate because many Baby Boomers will have the opportunity to stay in their own homes as they age.

Healthy aging is a primary goal of prescribing exercise medicine. The more successful aging adults are at adhering to the exercise physiologist's prescription for productive aging, they will be able to reduce the likelihood of disability and the need for long-term care (Rowe & Kahn 1998). Successful aging will also position the elderly and their lifestyle choices to be more productive members of society. This is important because aging of populations is rapidly increasing worldwide. It is a foregone conclusion that adults must start caring for themselves. After all, keep in mind that life is about more than going to work, getting a paycheck, raising a family, and doing what one can to be happy (although obviously important and expected as adults). Life is also about being responsible as an adult to maintain one's health and well-being so that life can be enjoyed and thoroughly lived.

---

**BOX 4.5   THE FUTURE OF OLDER ADULTS AND REALIZING THEIR FULL POTENTIAL.**

As the research points out, the decrease in mental and physical ability so commonly associated with aging is only loosely related to a person's chronological age. Yet a person's life course is almost without except driven by a sedentary lifestyle that sets the stage for multiple mental and physical health problems. Aging should the opportunity to continue living a great life without health problems, high costs of medical issues, and a decrease in lifespan. To help increase the likelihood of successful aging, physical activity and good nutrition can have powerful benefits for health and well-being that will allow for a dignified life with opportunities for continued personal growth.

Estimates by the Congressional Budget Office indicate that long-term care expenditures were more than $120 billion in 2000, with ~60% of the expenses covered by the public sector. Private insurance covered 1% of the long-term care costs, which out-of-pocket expenses accounted for essentially all of the balance. CBO indicated that total long-term care expenses will increase at a rate of 2.6% per year about inflation over the next 30 years, to $154 billion in 2010, $195 billion in 2020, and $270 billion in 2030.

This idea is linked to the concept of active aging, whereby society and individuals optimize opportunities to enhance personal health and quality of life. This means that society not only does what it can to help with economic and social services on behalf of the aging process but also that adults do what they can to prevent and decrease their personal and financial burden of chronic diseases, disabilities, and premature death. Protecting and promoting health by both personal means and social services are two primary responsibilities of each individual, regardless of his or her age and/or status.

Engaging in regular exercise has many physical and mental benefits, including increased longevity (especially in adults older than 60 years). The benefits are multiple, particularly in the decrease of anxiety and depression while increasing cognitive function and self-esteem, developing muscle strength, endurance, and flexibility, preventing disease, and reducing the risk of coronary heart disease, stroke, and diabetes. Among adults who engage in regular physical activity that includes resistance training, there is a decrease in the relative risk of developing functional limitations and the risk of falls.

## Vital Directions for Health Care

While it is clear that the doctorate-prepared exercise physiologists are driven to pursue research and publishing, the primary goal of the non-doctorate exercise physiologists is to prescribe exercise medicine. Research provides the academic exercise physiologists with a job with a good salary while the entrepreneurial approach to exercise medicine is the inroad to a credible job after college for the Bachelor of Science and the Master of Science prepared exercise physiologists.

Exercise medicine is an important direction for exercise physiologists. In fact, it is the opportunity for the profession of exercise physiology to help adults throughout the United States. When properly prescribed by exercise physiologists, exercise is medicine that helps to prevent and treat obesity, chronic diseases, and disabilities. In so doing, exercise medicine can help offset the U.S. $2.7 trillion on a healthcare system that treats disease and $350 billion spent annually on prescription drugs (Metzl 2013).

---

**BOX 4.6   THE NEED FOR PREVENTIVE HEALTH CARE IS CRITICAL FOR BETTER HEALTH AND LONGEVITY.**

Health care should be driven by preventive measures to increase health, well-being, and longevity. It should not be the outcome of spending trillions of dollars on expensive equipment, medications, and status quo, which raises the question: Why aren't the medical doctors dispensing the drug of exercise? The research worldwide supports the fact that low fitness and the lack of regular exercise is a major public health epidemic that needs correcting. Obesity itself is a major health concern that is responsible for high healthcare costs.

Rowe et al. (2016) said, "our health care system is unprepared to provide the medical and support services need for previously unimagined numbers of sick older persons, and we are not investing in keeping people healthy into their highest age." Despite increased awareness for new models of care, the same is also true for the exercise physiology academic major that should address society's aging issues in the curriculum. The ideal situation is one in which the physiology of healthy aging is incorporated within the exercise physiology course content, with a more comprehensive physiological assessment plan on aging in the exercise physiology laboratory. New lectures on caring for older adults in such neglected areas as health promotion and prevention, long-term care, and palliative care should be developed to help ensure high-quality services to the growing elderly population.

Presently, the number of ASEP Board-Certified Exercise Physiologists prepared is too few to sustain the effort that is needed to prevent avoidable issues associated with aging. The reasons are many, but a prominent impediment is the reluctance of academic exercise physiologists to do the work that is required to convert exercise science, kinesiology, and human performance academic degree majors to exercise physiology by title and curriculum content. Thus, the lack of a widespread adoption of the ASEP agenda allows for the mix of academic majors to continue as they have been for decades. The failure to acknowledge the value of the ASEP accreditation of academic majors leaves the students deficient in the evaluation and management of unique healthcare needs and treatment preferences of older adults.

Exercise physiology students at the doctorate level are confused when they find out that the academic major does not require them to take a course that lays out the management of common geriatric problems. This is a legitimate concern that is seldom discussed in academia, especially since it stands to impact the caliber of the students' education. Without a thorough understanding of the healthcare problems faced by older adults, students are at a distinct disadvantage.

Exercise physiology as a healthcare profession continues to suffer as a result of its failure to require competencies in the recognition, prevention, and management of frailty in older adults. Under the old-style doctorate training, students are expected to learn the acute responses and chronic adaptations of the body to exercise with very little understanding of the aging process. Learning just physiology as a rite of passage to sports training without learning the physiology and anatomy of chronic diseases, disabilities, and aging is a problem that requires significant reform. The students' education and career after college have suffered because they have limited knowledge of how to treat older patients.

The ASEP perspective is that exercise physiologists need training in all settings where older adults received care, including assisted living facilities, nursing homes, and patients' homes. As a starting point, exercise physiologists should demonstrate their competence in the care of frail older adults by passing the ASEP Board Certification exam (also known as the "Exercise Physiologist Certified" exam, EPC) (American Society of Exercise Physiologists 2019b). At some point, the majority of older adults will come face to face with illness and/or disability. With the decline in their health and functional status, it is important that they are helped by qualified professionals, such as the ASEP Board-Certified Exercise Physiologist.

---

**BOX 4.7  QUALITY OF LIFE IS IMPROVED BY THE ASEP EXERCISE MEDICINE PROFESSIONAL.**

Given that exercise is medicine, then it should be obvious that exercise medicine should be prescribed by Board-Certified Exercise Physiologists.

---

Since 1997, the professional advancement of exercise physiology has been made possible because of the existence of the profession-specific American Society of Exercise Physiologists. The ASEP leadership, like the leaders of the American Physical Therapy Association, understands the differences between a generic organization and a profession-specific organization. That is why they created long-term strategic priorities that benefit the membership and not the organization. The leadership of ASEP is responsible for ensuring the welfare of the membership before it works to ensure its longevity and financial base, even if it means doing so while using uncommon thinking and behavior.

---

**BOX 4.8  EXERCISE MEDICINE IS TAUGHT BY EXERCISE PHYSIOLOGISTS.**

Exercise physiology has emerged as a scientific education that first and foremost is responsible for the teaching and implementation of exercise medicine.

---

The idea that exercise physiologists do not need to teach about aging, advanced illnesses, and end-of-life care and issues is a weak argument, as is the idea that membership in generic organization is as good as membership in a profession-specific organization. Many exercise physiologists have little knowledge of how vulnerable elderly frail adults are compared to elderly non-frail adults. One wonders if they realize just how unprepared they are to work with clients and/or patients to prevent and treat chronic diseases and disabilities. My concern is with the academic exercise physiologists. Do they understand the language of frail older Americans sufficiently to qualify as healthcare professionals? Also, are they willing to work with the leadership of ASEP to ensure appropriate training and certification to advance the exercise physiologists' standards of care for patients with a chronic disease, disability, and frailty?

## Geriatric Exercise Physiology

The current number of exercise physiologists certified by ASEP is expected to increase in the coming years, which is critical to prevent, or at least mitigate, the expected shortage of gerontological nurses in the United States. But, unfortunately, just as most RNs have little to no training in gerontological nursing (Rosenfeld et al. 1999), the shortage of geriatric exercise physiologists is even more acute. The current number of exercise physiologists in long-term care settings is not known, but there is little doubt that the number is close to 0%. Other professionals also have a similar shortage of geriatric-educated healthcare professionals (Box 4.9).

---

**BOX 4.9   THE SHORTAGE OF GERIATRIC HEALTHCARE PROFESSIONALS.**

Less than 10% (i.e., 14 of the 145) U.S. medical schools require a geriatrics course, and less than half of 1% of the medical faculty are geriatric specialists. Only 720 of 200,000 pharmacists in the United States have geriatric certification. There are ~2,400 geriatric psychiatrists in the United States, but at least 5,000 are needed to deal with the mental healthcare problems of older adults.

—Bennett, JA, Flaherty-Robb, MK. (2003). Issues Affecting the Health of Older Citizens: Meeting the Challenge. *Online Journal of Issues in Nursing.* 8;1–11 [Online]. www.nursingworld.org/MainMenuCategories/ANAMarketplace/ANAPeriodicals/OJIN/TableofContents/Volume82003/No2May2003/OlderCitizens HealthIssues.aspx

—Merck Institute of Aging & Health and The Gerontological Society of America. (2002). *The State of Aging and Health in America* [Online]. www.aging society.org/agingsociety/publications/state/index.html

---

Interestingly, not only do many Americans view aging with fear and trepidation but also the healthcare-oriented educational programs are apparently not interested in giving priority to providing academic time to better understand the fear of aging. Therefore, it is common knowledge that the words "aging" and "nursing home" are associated with suffering, isolation, and fear in the minds of most middle-aged and older adults (Bennett & Flaherty-Robb 2003).

This lack of understanding of "what is aging" and "how to go about successful aging" is a problem throughout America if not the world. A major factor that has resulted in such thinking is the poor motivation to make personal health-oriented decisions about the best way to go live a healthy life and respect the aging process for what it is (e.g., the physical changes that ultimately are associated with a decrease in function and structure). Hopefully, the future of aging will become a topic of increased interest without fear or grief. Good health can be sustained longer than most Americans understand if only they would engage in an exercise medicine program that is good for both the mind and the body.

The challenge before exercise physiologists is not to be a copycat of the present-day healthcare providers, but rather to help the elderly aged 70 years and above who are not frail and those who are frail to enjoy an increase in their quality of life as well as decrease social and family burden. This is a critically important objective since the number of older adults is projected to be 70 million by 2030 and 82.3 million by 2040.

Also, of importance is the fact that by 2040 there will be 14.6 million adults 85 years of age and older. The 65 and older population is projected to increase between 80 million and 90 million by 2050, and the 85 and older population is projected to increase to ~21 million (Federal Interagency Forum on Aging-Related Statistics 2004). Many of these adults will experience a decline and deterioration of functional properties at the cellular, tissue, and organ level, which will result in a loss of homeostasis and adaptability to internal and external stressors with an increase in the likelihood of disease and mortality (Fedarko 2011).

Physical exercise (i.e., exercise medicine) is important for people of all ages to avoid if possible or at least minimize the negative effects of frailty. Exercise medicine improves health and well-being by decreasing the risk of many health problems associated with the elderly frail adults. The medical and scientific communities acknowledge that exercise is medicine because it decreases the risk of chronic diseases, impairments, and disabilities as well as resulting in psychological and cognitive benefits, and yet so few adults engage in aerobic and/or resistance training exercises.

---

### BOX 4.10   WHAT IS THE PERCENT OF ADULTS WHO ENGAGE IN REGULAR EXERCISE?

In regard to the 2008 Federal Physical Activity Guidelines, as reported in the *Federal Interagency Forum on Aging-Related Statistics, Older Americans 2016: Key Indicators of Well-Being*, only 12% of the adults 65 and older in 2014 participated in leisure-time aerobic and muscle-strengthening activities, and the percentage of older adults who met the guidelines decreased with age, ranging from 15% among adults who were 65 to 74 years old to 5% among adults aged 85 and over. However, although only 12% of the adults aged 65 and over met the guidelines for both aerobic and resistance training in 2014, 37% met the guidelines for aerobic exercise and 17% met the muscle-strengthening requirement for that year.

---

Between now and the end of the century, there will be more thin and weak adults with little to no energy. They will be easily tired and so their walking speed will be extremely slow. They are the elderly adults who usually suffer from three or more of the five following symptoms: unintentional weight loss of 10 or more pounds within the past year, muscle loss, a feeling of fatigue, a slow and unsteady walking speed, and a low level of physical activity. These age-related changes in muscle mass and diminished physical tolerance mean that an increased number of elderly people need only a minor illness or a fall to render them ill or hospital dependent (Box 4.11).

---

### BOX 4.11   FRAIL ADULTS AND PREDICTING THE END OF LIFE.

Putting a frail person in the hospital is often the beginning of the end.

---

It has become accepted that the diagnosis of frailty is increasingly linked to older adults and the end of life. So, why aren't adults or patients with frailty more aware of the importance of the corrective measures (i.e., palliative care) to engage in the appropriate intervention? Clearly, frailty is linked to a number of adverse outcomes, such as a decrease in strength, endurance, physiologic function, falls, disabilities, delirium, and mortality. Stow et al. (2018) indicate that the timely recognition of these outcomes is certainly a strong indicator of a life-limiting diagnosis, given the frailty trajectory in the last 12 months of life.

Timely recognition of the end-of-life phase is fundamental to the health care of older adults. Fortunately, there will be in the near future an increase in care provided by geriatric exercise physiologists who can improve the health and fitness of patients with frailty. Geriatric exercise physiologists will provide clients and patients with support during their diagnosis and treatment periods.

They will also help improve the outcomes, decrease the symptoms associated with frailty, and manage unfortunate side effects of severe comorbidities. The exercise itself will play an important role in improving psychological health, as well as decreasing the loss of the musculoskeletal system experienced by frail older adults.

Although recommending regular exercise should be encouraged by the older adults' physicians to deal with aging and sedentariness, physicians are not likely to offer advice on exercise training in the frail elderly population (Damush et al. 1999). Thus, it is important that exercise physiologist with an interest in geriatric exercise medicine gives advice to older adults about how to exercise and do so safely. They can do this as part of the treatment program in their exercise medicine clinics or as part of the total care of all clients and/or patients regardless of age.

## Final Thoughts

Among the ~329 million Americans in the United States, there will be an increase in the frail older adults who are highly susceptible to physical injury and infection (Fried et al. 2001). In fact, by 2030, there will be more than 70 million older Americans (*American Geriatrics Society* 2019), especially in California (39.5 million) and Texas (27 million). The most populous city in the United States is New York (8.5 million) (United States Population 2019).

Without question, the projected life expectancy will continue to increase with frail older adults who have impairments in balance, strength, mobility, endurance, physical activity, and cognition (Ferrucci et al. 2004). Hence, while there isn't any doubt, every exercise physiologist in the United States will need an ASEP accredited academic degree in the scientific concepts underlying the prescription of exercise medicine.

---

**BOX 4.12   ASEP AND GERIATRIC HEALTH CARE.**

It is the desire of the ASEP leadership that ASEP Board-Certified Exercise Physiologists with an interest in geriatric health care improve the health, functional fitness, and quality of life of older adults. The leadership believes that doing so will help ensure that older adults will continue to live a meaningful life as they age.

---

# References

*American Geriatrics Society.* (2019) [Online]. www.americangeriatrics.org/about-us

*American Society of Exercise Physiologists.* (2019a). *Accredited Programs* [Online]. www.asep.org/professional-services/accredited-programs/

*American Society of Exercise Physiologists.* (2019b). *Exercise Physiologist Certified* [Online]. www.asep.org/epc-online/epc-missionpurpose/

Bault, MW. (2012). *Americans with Disabilities: 2010.* Washington, DC: U.S. Census Bureau, U.S. Department of Commerce.

Bennett, JA, Flaherty-Robb, MK. (2003). Issues Affecting the Health of Older Citizens: Meeting the Challenge. *Online Journal of Issues in Nursing.* 8;1–11 [Online]. www.Nursing world.org/Main MenuCategories/ANAMarketplace/ANAPeriodicals/OJIN/TableofContents/Volu me82003/No2M ay2003/OlderCitizensHealthIssues.aspx

*Congressional Budget Office.* (1999). *CBO Memorandum: Projections of Expenditures for Long-Term Care Services for the Elderly.* Washington, DC.

Cook, C. (2012). This Is Not Your Parents' Aging Experience: How Geriatric Care Managers Can Leverage Their Knowledge and Know-How and Network to Respond to Baby Boomer Trends. *Journal of Aging Life Care.* 22(2);5–9.

Damush, T, Stewart, A, Mills, K, King, A, Ritter, P. (1999). Prevalence and Correlates of Physician Recommendations to Exercise Among Older Adults. *Journal of Gerontology: Medical Sciences.* 54A;423–427.

Faureault, MM, Smith, KE. (2004). A Primer on the Dynamic Stimulation of Income Model, DYNA-SIM3. Washington, DC: *Urban Institute* [Online], www.urban. org/UploadedPDF/410961_Dyna-sim 3Primer.pdf

Fedarko, NS. (2011). The Biology of Aging and Frailty. *Clinical Geriatric Medicine.* 27(1);27–37.

*Federal Interagency Forum on Aging-Related Statistics.* (2004). *Older Americans 2004: Key Indicators of Well-Being. Federal Interagency Forum on Aging-Related Statistics.* Washington, DC: U.S. Government Printing Office [Online]. https://agingstats.gov/docs/PastReports/2004/OA2004.pdf

*Federal Interagency Forum on Aging-Related Statistics.* (2016). *Older Americans 2016: Key Indicators of Well-Being. Federal Interagency Forum on Aging-Related Statistics.* Washington, DC: U.S. Government Printing Office. August 2016 [Online]. https://agingstats.gov/docs/Latest Report/Older-Americans-2016-Key-Indicators-of-Well Being. pdf

Ferrucci, L, Guralnik, JM, Studenski, S, et al. (2004). Designing Randomized, Controlled Trials Aimed at Preventing or Delaying Functional Decline and Disability in Frail, Older Persons: A Consensus Report. *Journal of the American Geriatrics Society.* 52(4);625–634.

Fried, LP, Tangen, CM, Walson, J, et al. (2001). Frailty in Older Adults: Evidence for a Phenotype. *Journal of Gerontology A: Biological Science and Medical Science.* 56(3);146–156.

Knickman, JR, Snell, EK. (2002). The 2030 Problem: Caring for Aging Baby Boomers, HSR: *Health Services Research.* 37(4);849–884.

*Merck Institute of Aging & Health and The Gerontological Society of America.* (2002). *The State of Aging and Health in America* [Online]. www.agingsociety.org/agingsociety/publica tions/state/index.html

Metzl, JD. (2013). The Exercise Cure: How Can We Motivate People to Take a Free, Safe, Magic Pill? *Slate* [Online]. https://slate.com/technology/2013/12/exercise-to-prevent-cure-or-treat-disease-cancer-heart-disease-inflammation.html

Redfoot, D, Feinberg, L, Houser, A. (2013). The Aging of the Baby Boom and the Growing Care Gap: A Look at Future Declines in the Availability of Family Caregivers. *AARP Public Policy Institute.* 85;1–12.

Rowe, J, Kahn, RL. (1998). *Successful Aging.* New York, NY: Pantheon.

Rosenfeld, P, Bottrell, M, Fulmer, T, Mezey, M. (1999). Gerontological Nursing Content in Baccalaureate Nursing Programs: Findings From a National Survey. *Journal of Professional Nursing.* 15(2);84–94.

Rowe, JW, Berkman, L, Fried, L, Fulmer, T, Jackson, J, Naylor, M, Novelli, W, Olshansky, J, Stone, R. (2016). *Preparing for Better Health and Health Care for an Aging Population*. Discussion Paper, Vital Directions for Health and Health Care Series. National Academy of Medicine. Washington, DC.

Stow, D, Matthews, FE, Hanratty, B. (2018). Frailty Trajectories to Identify End of Life: A Longitudinal Population-Based Study. *BMC Medicine*. 16(171);1–7.

*United States Population*. (2019) [Online]. http://worldpopulationreview.com/countries/united-states-population/

# 5

# THE PRESCRIPTION FOR AGING

What is the answer to the frailty problem? Is it taking a pill or is it exercise? The answer is obvious. Ask anyone and you get the same response. Pill or exercise, which one are you interested in? Without question, both the pill and exercise can help prevent stroke, heart disease, obesity, diabetes, and some kinds of cancers. Why not take the pill? It is easy to do. No sweat or time is taken to go for a walk. If the bones are weak, take a bone pill. If the muscles need to be stronger, take a muscle pill. Today, there is a pill for every ache, pain, and desire. Do you want to increase your attention span? Take a pill. How about your appetite? Do you find yourself with little desire to consume food or the right kinds of food? Take a pill. Well, there is just one catch. There is no such magic pill for each of these concerns. The answer to all of these concerns is exercise (Shaw 2004).

When I was in my second year of college, my father told me that exercise helps to protect against many different diseases, and yet it was clear then and still is today that the majority of the population isn't interested in exercising. Essentially every person I know has turned a blind eye to the protective effects of regular exercise. They are not interested in the epidemiological research, regardless of whether they are highly educated professionals or otherwise. They may actually believe that exercise is good for them, but they refuse to stop watching television, get out of the chair and go for a walk. If you share with them the smallest bits of information about why exercise is good for virtually every tissue in the body, more often than not they will leave the room while saying: "I am healthy. I don't need 30 min of walking or whatever type of PE you are doing today. By the way, yesterday I did a few things around the house."

It is a common fact that 75% of the population of the United States do not meet the minimum expectation of 30 minutes of walking a day to accumulate 150 min·wk$^{-1}$ or even 50 min·d$^{-1}$ 3 times·wk$^{-1}$ (such as Monday, Wednesday, Friday (MWF)). Yet, once again, there is irrefutable evidence that exercise (such as walking, bicycling, tennis, golf, and swimming) is good for a variety of mind and body health reasons, regardless of the person's age, gender, physical abilities, and medical conditions (Boone 2013). Without exercise as the means of burning calories, the outcome is obvious. Two-thirds of Americans are either overweight or obese, which increases their risk for cardiovascular disease, type 2 diabetes, and some cancers. Young children and teenagers are also prone to not exercise, and they too are developing diabetes with a predictable decrease in their lifespan.

DOI: 10.4324/9781003119920-7

The problem is that, regardless of age, there is an obvious imbalance in the energy consumed versus the energy expended (i.e., too much food consumed and too little exercise). This arrangement is not the right prescription for aging, and it does not matter where the calories come from (i.e., consuming too much food at every meal and/or eating fast-food meals rather than a balance caloric meal). Consuming too many calories is simply not a good thing to do. The calories must be used by the body, as when engaging in physical activity or otherwise the outcome is obvious. A lifestyle defined by a high caloric intake results in an increase in body mass. It isn't complicated why obesity is so common, especially when sedentary behavior is neglected.

The facts are clear. Too much sitting, watching TV, working on the computer, or looking at the phone increases the risk of cardiovascular disease. Everyone should be aware that people are spending more and more time doing sedentary activities. This is one side of the coin. The other side is all about exercising. Both sides of the coin must be addressed with precision to reduce the obesity problem in the United States and throughout the world (Shaw 2004). Otherwise, without exercising, the risk of being type 2 diabetic is high, especially in conjunction with obesity.

The Centers for Disease Control and Prevention (CDC) report that more than 30 million Americans have diabetes, and another 84 million adults have prediabetes. A person with diabetes is at a very high risk of blindness, kidney failure, and amputation of a toe, foot, or leg. This is a major problem, given that in the last 20 years, adults diagnosed with diabetes have tripled in the U.S. population among older adults who are overweight (*Centers for Disease Control and Intervention* 2019).

Research shows that dysfunction, disabilities, and diseases are linked with aging. It is important that the role of physical activity (i.e., bodily movement produced by the contraction of skeletal muscle that increases energy expenditure) is understood to benefit older adults, especially since 90% or more of diabetes is "adult-onset" or the type 2 form of the disease that can be prevented or delayed by regular exercise. But how often have you heard someone say, "I am too old to exercise. Forget it. I plan to kick back in my lazy-chair and take a long nap."

---

**BOX 5.1   PHYSICAL ACTIVITY IMPROVES BLOOD GLUCOSE CONTROL.**

"Although physical activity (PA) is a key element in the prevention and management of type 2 diabetes, many with this chronic disease do not become or remain regularly active. High-quality studies establishing the importance of exercise and fitness in diabetes were lacking until recently, but it is now well established that participation in regular PA improves blood glucose control and can prevent or delay type 2 diabetes, along with positively affecting lipids, blood pressure, cardiovascular events, mortality, and quality of life. Structured interventions combining PA and modest weight loss have been shown to lower type 2 diabetes risk by up to 58% in high-risk populations."

—Colberg, SR, Sigal, RJ, Fernhall, B, et al. (2010). Exercise and Type 2 Diabetes: The American College of Sports Medicine and the American Diabetes Association: Joint Position Statement. *Diabetes Care.* 33(12);147–167.

They are not interested in going for a 10- or 20-min walk or even riding a bicycle for 20 min. It is unfortunate that the earlier statement is very common among middle-aged and older adults. The truth is that exercise medicine helps to decrease the chance of developing a serious health condition (whether it is high blood pressure or diabetes). Also, when done correctly, exercise medicine is not dangerous.

Physical activity and exercise are important because both help older adults to age without chronic diseases and/or disabilities. As to how much exercise is needed to live a healthy life is easy to understand when adults are told that any amount of exercise is better than being sedentary. This is true even if the adult's physical status keeps him or her from achieving the recommended goals. Of course, the best approach to starting an exercise medicine program is to follow an "exercise prescription" with the guidance of an ASEP Board-Certified Exercise Physiologist to account for the adult's health status and functional capacity.

## The Aging Body

There was a time when everyone was young or middle-aged, but today life is much different. With just a little visual analysis, there is evidence of aging bodies in many ways that have not been thought about and/or considered before. While it is not possible without laboratory equipment to look at the aging body and see the changes in genes and biochemical processes along with the cellular changes and damage at the molecular level, aging is certainly associated with damage to the multiple systems (including the mitochondria that leads to the oxidation of low-density lipoproteins that is linked to atherosclerosis and coronary artery disease).

In the United States, aging is linked to more than 100,000 deaths each day, and ~67% of all deaths worldwide are due to aging. If it isn't death, then it is an increase in suffering from a multitude of medical conditions. The cost of the most common chronic medical conditions in the United States is close to $280 billion while the loss in productivity each year is ~$1 trillion (*Fight Aging: FAQ* 2019). Aging is very costly, in both dollars and quality of life. Yet the risk of dealing with age-related diseases and/or disabilities can be decreased for many people through regular exercise (i.e., exercise medicine) and dieting.

Hopefully, through new developments in scientific research in biotechnologies and the work of middle-aged "exercise active" individuals to prevent frailty and disease, living tomorrow and years thereafter with health and vigor will become reality. But, meantime, the benefits of exercise medicine are already a proven reality for living a better life without heart disease, dementia, diabetes, and many other age-related conditions. It is also important to manage stress, both physically and emotionally. After all, lifestyle choices have positive and negative effects on a person's chemistry. That is why meditation and the proper handling of mental stress throughout the day can add years of quality to an adult's life.

Aging is an ongoing disaster that is crippling older adults throughout the United States and throughout the world. It is a medical condition that takes joy from living and, strangely enough, society is not doing what it can in terms of exercise and diet to live a longer life without dying from the age-related conditions that decrease health and life expectancy. The clock is ticking. Either the causes of aging are better understood and middle-aged adults make significant personal changes to promote a longer and healthier lifestyle or they give in and accept the predictable decrease in longevity.

---

**BOX 5.2   A STARTING POINT FOR FAILING TO LIVE LONGER IS AN UNHEALTHY LIFESTYLE.**

It is unfortunate but true that continuing to live an unhealthy lifestyle predictably increases the negative effects of aging. By failing to adopt a better diet and exercise lifestyle, the increase in metabolic waste products decreases the ability to cope.

---

Although the human body is complex, both aging and quality of life are personal decisions to avoid as much as possible the accumulation of damage due to the failing of biological systems. How? Primarily by seeking the guidance and supervision of exercise physiologists trained in exercise medicine. Yes, as has been repeated many times in earlier chapters, frailty is a clinical geriatric syndrome caused by physiological deficits across multiple systems and exercise is medicine of choice. Thousands of scientific studies have demonstrated that the aging body can benefit greatly from even low-intensity exercise. Yes, exercise medicine at moderate intensity is known to decrease the risk of suffering from the common age-related diseases and disabilities. The bottom line, however, is that there isn't any significantly different health reason to engage in a higher intensity of effort.

---

**BOX 5.3   A REVOLUTION IN THE HEALTH BENEFITS OF EXERCISE IS UNDERWAY.**

It is well-known that as the population ages without living a healthy lifestyle, the prevalence and costs of musculoskeletal and cardiovascular diseases and disabilities are only going to increase. That is why knowledge of the body, how it functions, the effects of aging, and exercise medicine are important for research for exercise physiologists. The exercise physiologists' dedication to a cognitive mastery of important issues that undergird health, wellness, fitness, and longevity is consistent with using exercise as the primary prescriptive form of medicine to fight aging.

---

A critically important point to highlight in regard to the prescription of exercise medicine by exercise physiologists is not to extend life to a certain age point (e.g., living to 100 years of age). Rather, the objective is to promote a lifestyle that allows for the opportunity to live life more abundantly and, in particular, without the age-related decrease in muscle mass, strength, and functional quality of life. To not pursue the objective is to accept the sedentary lifestyle with a predictable loss of at least 5% of muscle mass per decade after 30 years of age.

Strangely enough, no one is asking the question: "Why is it that the typical middle-aged adult does not take part in a progressive resistance training program to help improve sarcopenia in as little as 2 weeks?" Part of the answer is this: The majority of adults perceive life in the context of working at a job, buying a home, raising a family, and paying bills. Aging is simply part of life, and too often there is little to no discussion about the necessity of young and older adults lifting weights (yet resistance training is important) and/or going for a 50-min walk 3 times·wk$^{-1}$.

## BOX 5.4   THE BENEFITS OF A PROGRESSIVE RESISTANCE TRAINING PROGRAM.

Strength-building exercises increase muscle strength, muscle protein synthesis, and muscle mitochondrial enzyme activity that ultimately decreases frailty in elderly adults by improving lean muscle mass and musculoskeletal function.

Living with sarcopenia is a common health problem that is seldom talked about or understood. Yet ~45% of older adults in the United States live with the age-related decrease in muscle mass. This is an important point because, in general, lean muscle mass approximates 50% of total bodyweight in young adults, and it is clear that it decreases with age to be about 25% of total bodyweight by 75 to 80 years of age (Short et al. 2004). This is a serious health and financial problem, given that the disability that results from sarcopenia accounts for ~$18 billion to $19 billion in direct medical costs.

Aside from the financial costs from the fourth to the approximately the seventh decade of life, the decrease in muscle mass means that the muscles are no longer as strong as they once were. As a result, there is an increased likelihood of falling that may cause a fracture and subsequent decrease in the ability to move about normally. The loss in musculoskeletal integrity with the predictable increase in bodyweight results in coordination problems that sets the stage for very slow movements with a decrease in metabolic rate, an increase in difficulty defending against pathogens due to an altered immune function, and a diminished quality of life.

Unless older adults stop the inevitable decrease in cognitive and physical health due to the lack of caring for their aging body, the prescription for frailty and major drugs dispensed by doctors will be met. Yet, while it is clear that all the medicines cannot prevent or reverse frailty as exercise medicine can, they may in fact actually cause many of the conditions associated with old age (e.g., forgetfulness, dementia, incontinence, and physical instability) (McTaggart 2010).

The scope of exercise physiology goes beyond the emphasis on the quick reach for the prescription pad to deal with the aging body and frailty. That is why it is important to emphasize a full and active lifestyle as the prescription for a long and healthy span of years. This is also why the ASEP leadership believes it is imperative that exercise physiologists as healthcare practitioners must acquire the knowledge necessary to preserve function and encourage healthy aging. This means avoiding the mindset that encourages an over-dependence on prescription drugs.

## BOX 5.5   IS IT BETTER TO TARGET PRE-FRAIL AND FRAIL OLDER ADULTS WITH DRUGS OR . . . ?

A lot of regular exercises, plenty of sunlight in the yard and working around the house, and good food as "the" prescription for long life without an increase in molecular and cellular damage, impairment in body functions, decrease in bone density, loss of lean muscle mass, poor vision, hearing, and cognition, and frailty.

The issue before ASEP exercise physiologists is to treat the weakness and decrease in walking speed of elderly adults as serious reasons for the increase in hospital use and costs (Garcia-Nogueras et al. 2017). Treatment begins with preserving function by starting an exercise program and improving nutrition to minimize the loss of skeletal muscle and strength associated with sarcopenia and frailty. However, as pointed out by Vellas and Sourdet (2017), "healthcare systems are not currently organized to deliver integrated care over the life course, but rather to identify and treat acute illness."

## Aging and Sarcopenia

Both healthcare delivery and policy must change to emphasize what is needed to avoid the progressive loss of muscle mass, strength, and physical function. This is necessary if healthcare professionals are to help younger individuals and the older adults to avoid the increase in drug treatment, caregiving costs, and the high risk of mobility disability that are related to the decrease in quality of life that is associated with sarcopenia (Goates et al. 2019).

---

**BOX 5.6 THE ECONOMIC IMPACT OF HOSPITALIZATIONS IN U.S. ADULTS WITH SARCOPENIA.**

"The total annual cost of hospitalizations for individuals with sarcopenia was USD $40.4 billion. . . . The total cost was higher in younger adults (USD $21.3 billion) compared to older adults (USD $19.1 billion)."

—Goates, S, Du, K, Arensberg, MB, Gailiard, T, Guralnik, J, Pereira, SL et al. (2019) Economic Impact of Hospitalizations in US Adults with Sarcopenia. *The Journal of Frailty & Aging.* 1–7 [Online]. Dx.doi.org/10.14293/jfa.2019.10

---

Sarcopenia is a significant public health issue, which is why it has been identified as a topic of concern to be examined by the United States 2020 Dietary Guidelines Advisory Committee (Goates et al. 2019). Young and older adults with chronic disease and extended periods of hospitalization are predisposed to the loss of muscle mass, strength, and physical function. Although sarcopenia is seldom identified as a major concern across age and race/ethnic groups, it is a costly public health problem.

In fact, according to Janssen et al. (2004), the hospitalization costs add up to US $40.4 billion annually for individuals with sarcopenia, which represents a major share of the total National Health Expenditures on hospital care (US $981.0 billion in 2014). Given the economic burden placed on the U.S. healthcare system by sarcopenia, there are important reasons to promote resistance training.

---

**BOX 5.7 IN ADDITION TO FLEXIBILITY TRAINING, EXERCISE MEDICINE IS A COMBINATION OF AEROBIC TRAINING AND RESISTANCE TRAINING.**

An important objective of the exercise medicine prescription by ASEP Board-Certified Exercise Physiologists is to reverse the decrease in muscle mass and poor functionality by engaging the client and/or patient in a progressive resistance training program to build the musculoskeletal system, which will also help in correcting the financial burden created by sarcopenia.

---

Although most researchers and healthcare professionals have thought of sarcopenia as an age-related loss of muscle mass and strength, Clark (2019) states that the problem may not be muscle atrophy per se but instead changes in the integrity of the nervous system. A different scientific point of view is that neurological and non-related muscle mass factors are responsible for the age-related decrease in muscle function. Hence, the primary factor responsible for muscle weakness in older adults is the reduced neural activation of the skeletal muscles.

It is reasonable to conclude that there are a number of changes with aging that also occur in the neuromuscular system. Any one change or a critical combination of two or more may contribute to the decrease in muscle size and function. For example, the decrease in the excitability of the corticospinal system has a negative effect on muscle function (Clark et al. 2011; Enoka et al. 2003). Clark (2011) indicates that the relationship between fat infiltration in muscle and dynapenia (i.e., the age-related decrease in muscle strength) contributes to muscle weakness, but the specifics are not fully understood.

Whether poor grip strength as one indication of frailty is an impairment of the neural drive to the muscles or the decrease in muscle mass and the decrease in muscle strength remains to be determined. What is important to remember is that the muscular system is responsible for the function of mobility (Fielding et al. 2011), and no magic pill has presented an improvement in strength and balance. Yet it is clear that bones become stronger, new capillaries throughout the body deliver more oxygen and nutrients, and the cognitive function is increased; all as the result of regular exercise.

These physiologic responses are the result of the magic pill, which is medicine delivered through the medium of exercise. Hence, exercise is the answer to skeletal muscle mass issues that allow for numerous physical and mental benefits (Box 5.8). Exercise is the medicine to reverse or mitigate frailty, enhance quality of life, and restore functioning in elderly frail adults or adults at risk of frailty.

---

**BOX 5.8  AGE-RELATED LOSS OF SKELETAL MUSCLE MASS AND FUNCTION CAN BE REVERSED.**

"It's never too late to treat frailty and recoup what you may have lost."

—Dr. Marian T. Hannan, Co-Director of the Musculoskeletal Research Center at the Institute for Aging Research at Harvard-affiliated Hebrew Senior Life.

---

Given that is the case, why is it that Shaw (2004) states that 75% of the population in the United States fail to meet the minimum recommendation for daily exercise of 30 min of walking? The obvious answer is that Americans love to think of themselves as being active and physically fit, but the reality is that many adults and children are overweight, unfit, and prone to chronic diseases. Why, because they are sedentary, which is an independent risk factor for coronary artery disease, hypertension, and a dozen other chronic diseases. The bottom line is that the longer the individuals, young and/or older adults, sit each day, the greater the risk of cardiovascular disease and sarcopenia. In essence, what this means is that the American lifestyle is not what it should be. But of course, this is also true for the rest of the world. Sedentary individuals are in love with watching TV and eating junk food. Being healthy has a price! Each person must cultivate the desire and will to be healthy. The quality of each person's life depends on his or her decision to do so.

Here are a few considerations that exercise physiologists can share with their clients and/or patients to help them take responsibility for their health: (a) develop the desire to live, which implies being healthy; (b) get with an exercise program; (c) avoid being caught up in quick-fix methods; (d) acknowledge the importance of personal control and self-discipline; (e) believe in yourself and do not let negative thinking deteriorate your state of mind; (f) be constructive and positive about exercise and critical thinking and don't worry; and (g) learn to be a friend to yourself (Boone 2002).

## Planning for the Future

While historically the elderly and frail could depend on family members to look after them, increasingly it is evident that is not the case. Today, help comes at a big cost from different healthcare businesses. Caregivers provide their services primarily in one of several ways. Either they go to an elderly adult's home to provide instructions and assistance in ways that are believed to help strengthen certain areas of the body that is believed to reduce pain, to increase range of motion, or to provide motivation to help with the frailty and physical decline. There are other types of assisted care facilities as well but at a steadily rising price a year (e.g., $100,000 in some nursing homes).

It is clear that if the elderly and the frail individuals are part of a fragmented family structure that is increasing every year along with the decrease in younger family members who were willing to help, then chances are that they are likely to experience an accelerated journey to debilitating frailty. Also, as a result of the fragmentation of the families, there is a growing concern about the quality of care and home-based out-of-pocket expenses for assistance (assuming the elderly adult has the financial resources). There are other concerns, too. In particular, since aging doesn't have to occur with frailty, why not avoid frailty and sarcopenia altogether? Why not avoid self-inflicted loss of skeletal muscle mass and strength? Why not stay strong into old age? Unfortunately, too many medical doctors treat their older patients with prescription drugs and seldom ever discuss the fact that growing older does not have to be a waste of a person's life.

Human beings are designed to move, to be active, to exercise, and live a lifestyle different from what has been accepted as the norm. Exercise medicine (i.e., aerobic training and resistance training among other training programs) is the answer to continuing to live with independence, quality of life, and longevity without assisted living facilities and drugs (Foster 2019). Aging with frailty is a losing battle, given the decrease in strength, mobility and balance problems, weak bones and fractures, weight gain/obesity and diabetes, and inability to cope with stressful conditions.

---

### BOX 5.9   MOST ADULTS NEED TO BE TOLD TO EXERCISE.

Board-Certified Exercise Physiologists are healthcare professionals who help their clients and patients to get up from reading, sitting at a desk, watching television, looking at Facebook, and going for a walk. Age-related muscle loss is a natural part of aging. After age 30 the third decade of life, adults lose 3% to 5% per decade, and most men will lose about 30% of their muscle mass during their lifetimes.

Obviously, aging without doing what one can to avoid frailty and sarcopenia is not a smart approach to life's health-related challenges. An age-related deficit that weakens normal function in the presence of one or more chronic diseases is consistent with the 10% or higher incidence of frailty in adults over 65 in the United States. Also, the longer adults live, the greater chance of becoming frail with poor outcomes that include disabilities, hospitalizations, and mortality. Given that frailty can be treated or prevented with regular exercise and diet means that exercise medicine is a serious healthcare inroad for ASEP Board-Certified Exercise Physiologists who can help adults face the new challenges of aging and their healthcare needs. Therefore, geriatric patients should make plans to consult ASEP exercise physiologists for a comprehensive physiologic and musculoskeletal assessment with an exercise prescription specific to tackle pre-frailty or frailty in its early stages, stop and/or delay its progression to disability, and (where indicated) assist with cognitive and psychosocial elements important in sustaining improvement and build resilience in building a new lifestyle.

## Final Thoughts

However difficult it is to grasp, it is nonetheless true every person will age. The question is this: "What can middle-aged adults do to help avoid aging poorly?" The evidence is clear, and it is not a radical departure from the lifestyle from which every person evolved. That is, increasing activity levels (such as walking, jogging, cycling, and swimming) will result in a healthier lifestyle. Hence, exercise is a medicine to live a healthier life for a longer period of time. There is strong evidence that exercise improves multiple systems throughout the body while inactivity and sitting for long periods of time day after day is the key to aging and the risk of chronic diseases, disabilities, and a short lifespan.

The "sit back and relax" mentality that characterizes an inactive lifestyle is highly correlated with one or more chronic diseases (i.e., a noninfectious health condition that cannot be spread from person to person). Obesity, in particular, is linked to type 2 diabetes mellitus, which is a leading cause of heart disease, stroke, kidney disease, and nerve damage. Hence, obesity is a major health problem that can be avoided by exercise (such as walking 30 min·d$^{-1}$ will decrease the risk of developing type 2 diabetes by 30 to 40%) (Shaw 2004).

The ASEP leadership is convinced that a new day is dawning for the profession of exercise physiology. They believe that although exercise physiologists will still be very interested in sports and human performance, there will also be an important emphasis on exercise medicine and aging. It is important that all academic exercise physiologists support ASEP and integrate an understanding of exercise physiology and exercise medicine as a required course in the exercise physiology major. A vision of this kind is timely, and it will make a professional difference in the students' education.

---

### BOX 5.10   EXERCISE MEDICINE IS PERTINENT TO THE PRACTICE OF EXERCISE PHYSIOLOGY.

Knowledge about healthy aging is vital for exercise physiologists. They will better understand muscle atrophy, muscle weakness, decrease in bone mineral density, thinning of articular cartilage, decreased cognitive processing, thickening of arterial walls, increased energy cost of breathing, decreased glucose tolerance, fewer T cell and B cell lymphocytes, and increased fibrosis in the colon. Thus, they will be in a better position to help their clients to adopt healthy practices to maximize fitness and prevent chronic diseases, falls, and disabilities.

## References

Boone, T. (2002). *The Power Within: The Integration of Faith and Purposeful Self-Care in the 21st Century*. Lewiston, NY: The Edwin Mellen Press.

Boone, T. (2013). *Introduction to Exercise Physiology*. Burlington, MA: Jones & Bartlett Learning.

Centers for Disease Control and Intervention. (2019). *Division of Diabetes Translation at a Glance* [Online]. www.cdc.gov/chronicdisease/resources/publications/aag/diab etes.htm

Clark, BC. (2011). Age-Related Changes in Motor Cortical Properties and Voluntary Activation of Skeletal Muscle. *Current Aging Science*. 4(3);192–199.

Clark, BC. (2019). Neuromuscular Changes with Aging and Sarcopenia. *The Journal of Frailty & Aging*. 8(1);7–9.

Colberg, SR, Sigal, RJ, Fernhall, B, Regensteiner, JG, Blissmer, BJ, Rubin, RR, Chasan-Taber, L, Albright, AL, Braun, B. (2010). Exercise and Type 2 Diabetes: The American College of Sports Medicine and the American Diabetes Association: Joint Position Statement. *Diabetes Care*. 33(12);147–167.

Enoka, RM, Christou, EA, Hunter, SK, Kornatz, KW, Semmler, JG, Taylor, AM, et al. (2003). Mechanisms that Contribute to Differences in Motor Performance between Young and Old Adults. *Journal of Electromyography and Kinesiology*. 13;1–12.

Fielding, RA, Vellas B, Evans, WJ, Bhasin, S, et al. (2011). Sarcopenia: An Undiagnosed Condition in Older Adults. Current Consensus Definition: Prevalence, Etiology, and Consequences. International working group on sarcopenia. *Journal of American Medical Directors Association*. 12;249–256.

*Fight Aging: FAQ*. (2019) [Online]. www.fightaging.org/faq/

Foster, GA. (2019). Aging Without Frailty: A Series (Part 2). *Make Aging Work* [Online]. https://makeagingwork.com/2019/02/11/aging-without-frailty-a-series-part-2/

Garcia-Nogueras, I, Aranda-Reneo, I, Pena-Longobardo, LM, et al. (2017). Use of Health Resources and Healthcare Costs Associated with Frailty: The FRADEA Study. *Journal of Nutrition and Healthy Aging*. 21(2);207–214.

Goates, S, Du, K, Arensberg, MB, Gailiard, T, Guralnik, J, Pereira, SL. (2019). Economic Impact of Hospitalizations in US Adults with Sarcopenia. *The Journal of Frailty & Aging*. 1–7.

Janssen, I, Shepard, DS, Katzmarzyk, PT, Roubenoff, R. (2004). The Healthcare Costs of Sarcopenia in the United States. *Journal of American Geriatric Society*. 52(1);80–85.

McTaggart, L. (2010). *A prescription for Old Age* [Online]. https://lynnemctaggart.com/a prescription-for-old-age/

Shaw, J. (2004). The Deadliest Sin: From Survival of the Fittest to Staying Fit Just to Survive: Scientists Probe the Benefits of Exercise—and the Dangers of Sloth. *Harvard Magazine*. March–April, 1–11 [Online]. https://harvardmagazine.com/2004/03/the-power-of-exercise

Short, KR, Vittone, JL, Bigelow, ML, Proctor, DN, Nair, KS. (2004). Age and Aerobic Exercise Training Effects on Whole Body and Muscle Protein Metabolism. *American Journal of Physiology-Endocrinology and Metabolism*. 286;92–101.

Vellas, B, Sourdet, S. (2017). Prevention of Frailty in Aging. *The Journal of Frailty & Aging*. 6(4);174–117.

# 6

# THE OLDER POPULATION

## What Is the Answer?

Frailty, sarcopenia, disability, and chronic diseases are increasing dramatically in the United States. The effects of the baby boom generation are evident throughout the population. The Administration on Aging has indicated that the U.S. population aged 65 and older increased by 40 million in 2010, which was a 15% increase in one decade, and it is expected to increase to 55 million (a 57% increase) by 2020 and will almost double (i.e., Americans over the age of 65) in a 30-year period (*Aging in Motion* 2018; *Administration on Aging* 2012).

Adults aged 90 and older are the fastest-growing segment in the United States, and it is expected to quadruple in size from 2010 to 2050 (He & Munchrath 2011). The increase in older adults means that frailty, functional decline, and disability are on the rise in America and, of course, this is true in countries throughout the world. Also, with the advancing age, there will be an increase in chronic diseases. In fact, 45% of the population or 133 million Americans have at least one chronic disease, which increases to 85% for adults aged 90 and older (He & Munchrath 2011).

Given the severity of being frail, "what is being done" to correct for the increase in health problems? This is an important question because millions of adults are institutionalized and admitted to long-term care facilities since they are not able to function at home due to their decreased mobility. The cost of health care is in the billions of dollars (Janssen et al. 2004; Thompson 2007). Given that both frailty and the healthcare costs continue to rise, what is the solution? Whatever the answer may be, without question it will involve exercise physiologists as credible healthcare professionals.

The frailty problem is real, and it needs help and support from organizations that have a strong educational emphasis on exercise physiology. Understanding just how serious the problem is, the work of the ASEP organization in pushing for an undergraduate accredited degree in exercise physiology will help. In particular, once the students complete the program, they are not required but encouraged to sit for the ASEP Board Certification exam. Upon passing the exam, they will earn the professional title, Board-Certified Exercise Physiologist with the academic training to prescribe exercise as medicine (i.e., exercise medicine).

Looking to the future, the ASEP exercise physiologists will be among the key healthcare professionals to treat frailty in the elderly adult population and their loss of physiological and

DOI: 10.4324/9781003119920-8

functional independence. Their exercise medicine healthcare practice will encompass the development of treatments and interventions to improve functional aerobic capacity, muscle strength, power, and endurance, as well as independence of the aging population (i.e., the syndrome of frailty, which is a good predictor of negative health outcomes). Without question, frailty can be prevented or treated with a safely prescribed exercise medicine program that consists of evidence-based aerobic exercise, resistance training (i.e., weight), and flexibility exercise program designed in a highly prescriptive manner for each individual adult.

## The Current Challenge

Is it that a treatment is only as good as it is an accepted part of the established medical system? Or, is a treatment viewed as credible if it comes from outside the traditional physician approach to health care? Although they are not 100% engaged in clinical practice, it is a fact that exercise physiologists are involved in the healthcare treatment of elderly frail adults to improve their quality of care and promote healthy aging. For this reason, exercise medicine implemented by ASEP exercise physiologist should not be challenged for quality or educational status.

Exercise medicine is logically the most effective treatment known for frailty and the most effective intervention to improve the health and well-being of frail older adults (Box 6.1). Frailty isn't the same as aging. Also, frailty is not a disease. Frailty is a way of living that is the result of disuse and loss of muscle mass as adults get older.

---

**BOX 6.1 THE EXERCISE MEDICINE PRACTICE BY EXERCISE PHYSIOLOGISTS IS CLEAR.**

There is excellent research that shows exercise medicine: (a) slows the aging process that impairs muscle function, physical activity, and walking; (b) promotes psychological and cognitive well-being; (c) decreases the risk of chronic diseases and disabilities; and (d) provides for increased independence, quality of life, and longevity.

---

The results are so overwhelmingly obvious that exercise medicine should be part of everyone's lifestyle at any age. Staying active physically is the equivalent of staying active mentally and, therefore, the opportunity to experience healthier aging into the older years. But, first, the current challenge is to get started. So, why isn't the medical community, especially the older adult's physician, sharing with the patient the role of the exercise physiologists in prescribing an exercise program? With due respect to medical doctors, the "basics" of the exercise medicine message is simply to get out of the chair, put down the book, phone, or computer, put on a good pair of walking shoes, and go outside and start one step at a time a walking program.

Young, middle-aged, older, and elderly adults should avoid physical inactivity at all cost. They should do at least 30 $min \cdot d^{-1}$ of either low- or moderate-intensity aerobic activity. But, if appropriate for the adult's physical condition, invite a friend to join in the walk. Start slowly, just for 10 min and take a few seconds of rest, and then make the commitment to complete the walk. Adults should also include resistance training exercises (i.e., muscle-strengthening activities) that involve all the major muscle groups throughout the body for at least 2 d·wk$^{-1}$ with either free weights or a machine (*U.S. Department of Health and Human Services* 2008). Be sure to breathe with a regular frequency and depth to avoid changes in blood pressure or developing an abnormal heart rhythm. Start with six to eight repetitions per exercise and build up to the second set.

It is interesting that the improvements in public health have resulted in an increase in life expectancy, and yet with the longer lifespan the adults have become frail older adults who are the main users of the medical and social care services. Between 2000 and 2050, the number of adults 60 years of age and older throughout the world is anticipated to double from 11% to 22%. This is an increase from 605 million to 2 billion adults aged 60 or older. During the same period, the number of older adults 80 years of age and over is projected to quadruple to 395 million (*U.S. Department of Health and Human Services* 2008).

The increase in older adults will also mean an increase in the number of frail older adults who will live with a decrease in physiological reserve plus a compromised capacity to live independently (Clegg et al. 2013), which means that frail older adults are key users of healthcare resources (Kojima et al. 2019). The problem is huge with decreased reserve and resistance to stressors with the world population projected to be greater than 7.5 billion individuals in 2020 with 1 billion to reach or exceed 65 years of age (Kinsella & Phillips 2005). The challenge of dealing with the healthcare concerns, the premature deaths, and all the disabilities will be essentially unmatched among the existing medical diseases, disabilities, and hospitalizations.

## A Collaborative Approach

Since frailty is associated with the elderly adult's genetic and environmental factors as well as several comorbid conditions, Spinewine et al. (2007) concluded that a collaborative approach should be used to identify, prevent, and treat frailty. In this regard, the ASEP perspective is not a complicated one. While specialty information from multidisciplinary medical professionals would no doubt provide geriatric screening and the identification of frailty, the work necessary to care for the elderly and the frail condition should be supervised by Board-Certified Exercise Physiologists. If there is the need for help from medical specialties such as geriatric medicine, geriatric psychiatry, palliative care, physical medicine, and rehabilitation, then certainly the management of the older adults' frailty would include coupling information from different sources.

Since physical inactivity and musculoskeletal weakness are primary concerns that are associated with frailty (Lally & Crome 2007), both highlight the importance of the exercise physiologist's exercise medicine prescription as a critical component of the management and prevention of frailty. Exercise medicine helps to correct the major components of the frailty syndrome, which are a decrease in physiological reserve and lean muscle mass (sarcopenia). It is reasonable that the initial screening for the identification of frailty by a physician will result in the referral of the frail adult to an exercise medicine clinic supervised by Board-Certified Exercise Physiologists. They will carry out the cardiorespiratory, musculoskeletal, and body fat evaluations to create the scientific and educational foundation for the exercise medicine prescription to slow the progression of the frailty syndrome. Overall, it will be important that the prescription is linked to a coordinated effort with other healthcare professionals to oversee an integrated nutritional, psychosocial, and pharmaceutical support and management.

Otherwise, it is critical that any adverse events such as falls, disabilities, fractures, and health care in response to delirium, malnutrition, and infections that often contribute to a slower adaptation to the exercise medicine prescription are cared for by regular provisions of physician visits and follow-up when indicated (Cohen et al. 2016; Purdy et al. 2012). Prevention should be implemented to promote positive aging and healthy behaviors (such as adequate nutrition and the reduction in alcohol and/or tobacco use) to prevent nutritional deficiencies and additional impairments (e.g., depression, negative cognitive outcomes, and a major loss of independence).

The age-related decrease in muscle mass, strength, and function (i.e., sarcopenia) is often accompanied by osteoporosis (a decrease in bone mass and strength) that can be a contributing factor in an older adult's increase in frail bones, falls, and fractures (Daly 2017). Hence, to avoid a loss of independence that decreases quality of life, physicians should work with exercise physiologists (via referrals) to help optimize muscle and bone health as well as functional capacity by targeting the muscle and bone connection through a regular walking program.

It should be pointed out that while Daly (2017) indicates there is the concern that regular walking may not be good enough to build strong bones. This is because walking is considered to be low impact exercise that results in less stress on the skeletal system and little to no increase in bone density. Brady (2017) disagrees up to a point (Box 6.2). For frail older adults just beginning a walking program, the impact of their foot hitting the ground will appear to be sufficient to produce stress and new bone formation.

Ma et al. (2013) reported that walking has little or no effect on preventing bone loss, which appears to be explained by the low impact loading forces that do not stimulate the osteocytes to cause an adaptive skeletal response. However, the ASEP leadership believes that walking is a serious healthcare intervention. To conclude that it isn't is premature. If exercise physiologists and other healthcare professionals are able to work together to get older and elderly men and women adults out of their comfortable chair and away from the TV to go for a walk, then why not? Also, not every older and elderly man or woman has bone density issues and, therefore, the idea that walking should not be recommended to decrease the likelihood of falls and fractures is highly questionable.

---

**BOX 6.2  THE LINK BETWEEN THE BONE-BUILDING BENEFITS AND WALKING.**

The key to the bone strengthening properties of walking is the amount of positive stress and impact created with the stride. Although regular walking does not appear to have significant effect on preservation of bone mineral density, fast walking or power walking does appear to have a positive influence on bone. It has been shown that walking 3 miles, 4 d·wk[-1], at a pace of greater than 3.8 mph, can increase leg muscle mass and preserve bone mineral density in postmenopausal women.

—Borer, KT, Fogleman, K, Gross, M, New, JM, et al. (2007). Walking Intensity for Postmenopausal Bone Mineral Preservation and Accrual. *Bone.* 41(4);713–721.

Equally important, since it is clear that many older adults may not be willing to engage in a supervised exercise program, why not consider a less structured and less demanding type of exercise to benefit the musculoskeletal system. Thus, in regard to the collaborative approach, it is important that exercise physiologists share their thoughts about frail elderly individuals walking, particularly as it relates to "sitting less and moving more" to build resilience and combat frailty.

*The Surgeon General's "Call to Action" to Promote Walking and Walkable Communities* (*Surgeon General.Gov* 2019) calls everyone to be physically active by creating a culture that supports these activities for people of all ages, sex, and abilities. Among aging adults, physical activity is associated with improvement in quality of life, emotional well-being, and positive mental health. Regular physical activity is also important for healthy aging and is likely to delay the onset of cognitive decline in older adults (*Physical Activity Guidelines Advisory Committee* 2008).

People can get these benefits through walking or by adding some brisk walking, which is also a necessary public health strategy for several reasons. Walking does not require special skills, facilities, or expensive equipment. For the most part, older adults are able to walk, and many elderly frail adults with disabilities are able to walk or move with assistive devices (such as a walker). There is also a low risk of injury whereby adults who are inactive become physically active because walking can be adapted to fit one's time and physical condition while:

- Improving blood pressure and blood sugar
- Reducing lipids in the blood
- Improving neuro-cognitive function
- Increasing the immune function
- Lowering the risk of heart disease
- Increasing bone density
- Improving range of motion and balance
- Lowering the risk of falls and bone fractures
- Increasing metabolism to improve gastrointestinal function
- Protecting against dementia and Parkinson's disease
- Extending functional independence
- Improving muscle strength, flexibility, and mobility
- Reducing widespread muscle pain

## Exercise: The Incredible Medicine

Hardly anyone is excited about taking drugs prescribed by physicians, but they do so anyway. Why? Because they were told that such-in-such drug lowers blood pressure or cholesterol, which is good if you are not interested in having a heart attack. After reading through the short list of benefits derived from exercising, why is it that the majority of teenagers and adults simply turn a deaf ear to the news that exercise is a miracle drug? Perhaps, simply stated, it is because exercise requires discipline more so than taking a pill to produce the benefits. Everyone is (or should be) interested in good health to live a long time. Longevity is important, but most adults are not interested in the work and discipline necessary to live a longer and healthier life. Yet it is clear that exercise slows aging, helps to reduce chronic pain, delays cognitive decline, and, therefore, improves brain health.

The "exercise medicine pill" does not require out-of-pocket expenses to experience its benefits. It is free to the person willing to go for a 30-min walk, lift some weights couple of times a week, and stretch the muscles of upper and lower limbs and lower back. In addition to these healthcare benefits, exercise decreases the risk of developing numerous chronic diseases, as well as decreases the risk for 13 types of cancer (Metzl 2018). Obviously, it is of crucial importance that individuals in public health and medicine start valuing and appreciating the role of exercise in the aging process. The hope is that physicians and exercise physiologists can work together to educate patients about exercise medicine and its relationship to specific health-related concerns.

Given the scientific findings that illustrate the age-related reduction in physiologic reserves from aging and inactivity, the sooner the medical community and society embrace exercise medicine, the better for all the obvious reasons (Box 6.3). In fact, as strange as it sounds to the majority, just 10,000 steps a day will help keep the doctor away. Nonetheless, it is true, and if the American people and everyone else worldwide would go for at least a 30-min or a 40-min walk 5 $d{\cdot}wk^{-1}$, physical inactivity would not be the fourth leading underlying cause of mortality. Also, there would be less health issues, frailty concerns, disabilities, and costly medical conditions.

---

**BOX 6.3  THE HEALTHCARE TREATMENT COST IN THE UNITED STATES.**

Think about it. The renowned sports medicine physician at the Hospital for Special Surgery in New York said, "Every year, Americans spend more than $3 trillion on health care, and most of that goes toward treating diseases." Rather expensive don't you think. Think with me again, regarding the fact that the United States ranks 43rd among the nations of the world in health and longevity.

—Metzl, JD. (2018). The Incredible Medicine of Movement. *The Science of Exercise: A True Medicine* [Online]. https://aktivmotkreft.no/wp-content/uploads/2018/09/exercise-intro.pdf

---

An adult may say to an exercise physiologist, "Will regular walking help me, being overweight and some may say obese?" "Yes." In fact, Michael J. Joyner, MD, is a physician and medical researcher at the Mayo Clinic in Rochester, Minnesota, with interest in exercise physiology and aging says it is important that overweight and obese adults start a walking program to reduce the risk of diabetes and high blood pressure.

Exercise is also a medicine that protects thinking skills. Godman (2018) points out in the Harvard Health Letter that this information comes at a critical time, especially since one new case of dementia is detected every 4 seconds globally, and by the year 2050, the estimate is that more than 115 million people will have dementia worldwide. The benefit of exercise is that it decreases insulin resistance, decreases inflammation, and stimulates the release of chemicals in the brain that affect the health of brain cells, the growth of new blood vessels in the brain, and the abundance and survival of new brain cells.

Exercise not only increases heart rate, which pumps more oxygen to the brain, but also helps in the release of hormones that provide an excellent environment for the growth of brain cells. Brain plasticity is stimulated by exercise that promotes the growth of new connections between cells in a wide array of important cortical areas of the brain. Research from UCLA by Molteni et al. (2004) supports this point by demonstrating that exercise increased growth factors in the brain, thus making it easier for the brain to grow new neuronal connections.

Unfortunately, very few adults who actually can benefit from regular exercise are seldom ever referred to as exercise physiologists. Even patients with cardiovascular disease are not helped as they should be. Boden et al. (2014) concluded it has been estimated that 20% to 30% of eligible patients receive referrals from their physicians to cardiac rehabilitation programs. Exercise medicine is a medical prescription that is seldom prescribed by the medical community. This is very alarming because the least fit throughout the United States and worldwide is missing out on the credible opportunity to improve the physiological changes of aging and disuse.

---

### BOX 6.4   THE POLYPILL OR EXERCISE.

"To date, there has not been any type of pharmacological intervention, i.e., a polypill that has provided the benefits to as many organ systems as regular physical activity."

—Bruning, RS, Sturek, M. (2014). Benefits of Exercise Training on Coronary Blood Flow in Coronary Artery-Diseased Patients. *Progress in Cardiovascular Diseases*. 57(5);443–453.

---

While the benefits of regular exercise for people of all ages are scientifically established, it is a serious problem that the medical community is not motivated to recommend exercise medicine. Therefore, the lack of exercise as a physician-ordered prescription continues to be a serious public health concern. Another concern is that many, if not the majority, of the adults are not interested in the exercise recommendations to increase exercise capacity and muscle mass. Muscle-strengthening (i.e., resistance training) exercises are particularly important for older adults, yet only a very small percent (perhaps 10%) of the adults 65 years and older actually adhere to the resistance training recommendation twice a week.

It is pastime to begin a public campaign concerning frailty and motivational steps to encourage regular exercise to decrease the negative effects of frailty. Older adults need to understand the power of the mind as a positive or negative influence on the role of exercise in their lives. For example, it isn't common for elderly people to think about or discuss among their friends how long will they live. This is especially true if they are living by themselves in a two-room assisted living facility with little to no meaningful social support. Loneliness may lead to the loss of motivation and purpose in most things in life (Sacha et al. 2017).

It is interesting that Sacha et al. (2017) indicated that an exercise and/or social program that deals only with the person's physiological needs is inadequate in motivating older adults to participate in life's activities. What was implied is that if an exercise medicine program exists, it is all about doing the exercise and little else. But, if the exercise is followed by an educational component with the purpose of understanding the role of the mind and the body and how they undergo positive physiological responses with regular exercise, the elderly person would very likely be a more active person. Social and educational interactions play an important role in keeping an interest in life and encouraging elderly subjects to think positively about living and exercising.

---

### BOX 6.5 THE BENEFITS OF A MULTICOMPONENT EXERCISE PROGRAM.

There isn't any question that exercise has beneficial effects on frail older adults. But exercise by itself is not enough. The exercise program should be 3 times·wk$^{-1}$ for 30 to 45 min·session$^{-1}$. There should be aerobic, resistance, flexibility, and balance training exercises with emphasis on better physiological health, stronger muscles, and balance. The program should include an educational component that teaches the basic responses and adaptations to the different types of exercise. There should be a positive psychological and cognitive component to the program with spiritual and existential concerns.

---

It is distressing to acknowledge that ~75% of older adults do not exercise at a high enough intensity to improve their health. In fact, Nied and Franklin (2002) indicate that only 16% of the adults 65 to 74 years of age complied with the 30 minutes or more of moderate exercise 5 or more days a week (*U. S. Department of Health and Human Services* 2008).

Understanding the geriatric problem society is faced with begins with the 2013 analysis of generational cohorts from the database of the National Health and Nutrition Examination Survey. The data show that regular exercise is significantly less frequent in the baby boomer generation than in the previous generation. Also, more than 50% of the baby boomers reported no regular exercise program as part of their lifestyle (King et al. 2013). In agreement, Prince (2014) pointed out, "These compelling epidemiologic data suggest that without a significant change in the overall physical activity level of the baby boomer generation, an epidemic of sedentarism-related burdens in our society will increase exponentially."

## Muscle Loss and Functional Decline

Sedentary behavior is a huge problem in our society. The question is this: What are the 45-, 65-, 75-, and 85-year-old men and women doing to keep themselves healthy? The short answer is "nothing," and this is true throughout world. Yet everyone wants to live longer and enjoy life to its fullest. Happiness and good health means everything to most people. But strange as it sounds, while an adult doesn't have to grow old and frail too, most will and many of them will experience functional decline.

Without living the life of a physical activity individual, most adults will experience issues of functional decline. It is common in older adults. In fact, it is so common that it begs the question: What are the healthcare professionals doing about it? Regardless of the older adult's education and/or financial status, what is he or she doing to avoid frequent falls, high blood pressure, cognitive impairments, insomnia, anxiety, depression, and sarcopenia? The evidence suggests that people worldwide are simply not motivated to identify a time period every other day to stop everything else and engage in a muscle-strengthening program.

Disability affects one in seven Americans who is either experiencing major difficulty in basic functional activities or still has some ability irrespective of muscle size (Colon-Emeric et al. 2013). The health conditions that may contribute to a functional disability are chronic diseases, neurologic issues, obesity, diabetes, fractures, and cognitive impairment, among others. The coexistence of two or more of these conditions often brings about an increase in functional decline (Tinetti et al. 1995). Here, the role of regular exercise is to increase the adult's capacity to respond to his or her challenges (Iwarsson 1996). Depending on the disability, there may also be the need for medical and surgical interventions to increase functional capacity as well as the consideration of various prosthetic devices and/or nutritional supplements (Colon-Emeric et al. 2013).

Aging is accompanied by a progressive decrease in muscle mass (sarcopenia) and muscle strength (dynapenia) that are important for safe locomotion (Kalyani et al. 2014). Age-related sarcopenia is a risk factor for disabilities, hospitalizations, and death in older frail adults (Fielding et al. 2011). Janssen et al. (2004) estimated that a 10% reduction in age-related lean muscle mass would result in a savings of $1.1 billion per year in healthcare costs in the United States. Hence, it is obvious that by decreasing the loss of muscle mass in older adults, the cost of health care would decrease and life would be easier with less falls and disabilities.

---

### BOX 6.6  AGE-RELATED LOSS OF LEAN MUSCLE MASS.

"Lean muscle mass generally contributes up to about 50% of total bodyweight in young adults, but decreases with age to be about 25% of total bodyweight by age 75–80 years."

—Kalyani, RR, Corriere, M, Ferrucci, L. (2014). Age-Related and Disease-Related Muscle Loss: The Effect of Diabetes, Obesity, and Other Diseases. *Lancet Diabetes & Endocrinology.* 2(10);819–829.

---

## Final Thoughts

It is clear that physical inactivity is a major contributor to age-related muscle loss and ultimately mortality. The World Health Organization (2013) reported that ~3.2 million deaths every year are attributable to the physical inactivity and the lack of resistance-based strengthening exercises. Fortunately, the ASEP Board-Certified Exercise Physiologists know exactly what to do to alter the negative effects of aging on metabolic, cardiovascular, and musculoskeletal functions throughout the body.

Exercise is a powerful medicine. Academic exercise physiology professors who are not seeking ASEP accreditation of their exercise physiology college major with the *American Society of Exercise Physiologists'* accrediting guidelines are neglectful of their professional responsibility, even to the point of unprofessional behavior. It is pastime to do what is right on behalf of the exercise physiology profession and their students. They must teach their students about the healthcare system and that they will graduate as ASEP healthcare providers who will be responsible for prescribing exercise as a drug.

The college professors who are exercise physiologists must start thinking about exercise physiology as a healthcare profession, updating the academic major, and seeking a better understanding of the future of exercise physiology and their graduating seniors as ASEP Board-Certified Exercise Physiologists as healthcare professionals. After all, exercise is medicine, and it would be a serious mistake to not understand the professional and legal responsibilities of exercise physiologists in prescribing exercise medicine.

## References

*Administration on Aging.* (2012). *A Profile of Older Americans 2010* [Online]. www.aoa.gove/aoaroot/aging_statistics/Profile/2010/16.aspx

*Aging in Motion.* (2018). *Frailty and Disability on the Rise in the US, But Where Is the Response?* [Online]. http://aginginmotion.org/frailty-and-disability-on-the-rise-in-the-us-but-where-is-the-response/

Boden, WE, Franklin, B, Berra, K, et al. (2014). Exercise as a Therapeutic Intervention in Patients With Stable Ischemic Heart Disease: An Underfilled Prescription. *American Journal of Medicine.* 127(10);905–911.

Brady, S. (2017). Walk Your Way to Stronger Bones. *Nurtured Bones* [Online]. https://nurturedbones.com/walk-your-way-to-stronger-bones/

Cohen, MS, Paul, E, Nuschke, JD, Tolentino, JC, et al. (2016). Patient Frailty: Key Considerations, Definitions and Practical Implications. *IntechOpen* [Online]. http://dx.doi.org/10.5772/64296

Colon-Emeric, CS, Whitson, HE, Pavon, J, Hoenig, H. (2013). Functional Decline in Older Adults. *American Family Physicians.* 88(6);388–394.

Clegg, A, Young, J, Iliffee, S, Rikkert, MO, Rockwood, K. (2013). Frailty in Elderly People. *Lancet.* 381(9868);752–762.

Daly, RM. (2017). Exercise and Nutritional Approaches to Prevent Frail Bones, Falls, and Fractures: An Update. *Climacteric.* 29(2);119–124.

Fielding, RA, Vellas, B, Evans, WJ, et al. (2011). Sarcopenia: An Undiagnosed Condition in Older Adults. Current Consensus Definition: Prevalence, Etiology, and Consequences. International Working Group on Sarcopenia. *Journal of American Medical Directors Association.* 12;249–256.

Godman, H. (2018). Regular Exercise Changes the Brain to Improve Memory, Thinking Skills. *Harvard Health Letter* [Online]. www.health.harvard.edu/blog/regular-exercise-changes-brain-improve-memory-thinking-skills-201404097110

He, W, Muenchrath, MN. (2011). *US Census Bureau, American Community Survey Reports, ACS-17, 90+ in the United States: 2006–2008.* US Government Printing Office, Washington, DC.

Iwarsson, S. (1996). Functional Capacity and Physical Environmental Demand. Exploration of Factors Influencing Everyday Activity and Health in the Elderly Population. *Scandinavian Journal of Occupational Therapy.* 3(3);139.

Janssen, I, Shepard, DS, Katzmarzyk, PT, Roubenoff, R. (2004). The Healthcare Costs of Sarcopenia in the United States. *Journal of the American Geriatric Society.* 52;80–85.

Kalyani, RR, Corriere, M, Ferrucci, L. (2014). Age-Related and Disease-Related Muscle Loss: The Effect of Diabetes, Obesity, and Other Diseases. *Lancet Diabetes & Endocrinology.* 2(10);819–829.

King, DE, Matheson, E, Chirina, S, et al. (2013). The Status of Baby Boomers' Health in the United States: The Healthiest Generation? *JAMA Internal Medicine.* 173(5);385–386.

Kinsella, KG, Phillips, DR. (2005). *Global Aging: The Challenge of Success.* Washington, DC: Population Reference Bureau, 60.

Kojima, G, Liljas, AEM, Iliffe, S. (2019). Frailty Syndrome: Implications and Challenges for Health Care Policy. *Risk Management and Healthcare Policy.* 12;23–30.

Lally, F, Crome, P. (2007). Understanding Frailty. *Postgraduate Medical Journal.* 83(975);16–20.

Ma, D, Wu, L, He, Z. (2013). Effects of Walking on the Preservation of Bone Mineral Density in Perimenopausal and Postmenopausal Women: A Systematic Review and Meta-Analysis. *Menopause.* 20;1216–1226.

Metzl, JD. (2018). The Incredible Medicine of Movement. *The Science of Movement: A True Medicine* [Online]. https://aktivmotkreft.no/wp-content/uploads/2018/09/exercise-intro.pdf

Molteni, R, Zheng, JQ, Ying, Z, et al. (2004). Voluntary Exercise Increases Axonal Regeneration from Sensory Neurons. *Proceedings of the National Academy of Sciences of the United States of America.* 101(22);8473–8478.

Nied, RJ, Franklin, B. (2002). Promoting and Prescribing Exercise for the Elderly. *American Family Physician.* 65;419–428.

*Physical Activity Guidelines Advisory Committee.* (2008). *Physical Activity Guidelines Advisory Committee Report.* Washington, DC: U.S. Dept of Health and Human Services.

Prince, DZ. (2014). *Exercise in the Elderly. American Academy of Physical Medicine and Rehabilitation* [Online]. https://now.aapmr.org/exercise-in-the-elderly-2/

Purdy, S, et al. (2012). *Interventions to Reduce Unplanned Hospital Admission. Bristol, United Kingdom: National Institute for Health Research* [Online]. www.bristol.ac.uk/media-library/sites/primaryhealthcare/migrated/documents/unplanned admissions.pdf

Sacha, J, Sacha, M, Sobon, J, Borysiuk, Z, Feusette, P. (2017). Is It Time to Begin a Public Campaign Concerning Frailty and Pre-Frailty? A Review Article. *Frontiers in Physiology.* 8(484);1–11.

Spinewine, A, Swine, C, Dhillon, S, et al. (2007). Effect of a Collaborative Approach on the Quality of Prescribing for Geriatric Inpatients: A Randomized, Controlled Trial. *Journal of the American Geriatrics Society.* 55(5);658–665.

*Surgeon General.Gov.* (2019). *Step It Up! The Surgeon General's Call to Action to Promote Walking and Walkable Communities: Executive Summary.* U.S. Department of Health & Human Services, Washington, DC [Online]. www.surgeongeneral.gov/library/calls/walking-and-walkable-communities/exec-summary.html

Thompson, DD. (2007). Aging and Sarcopenia. *Journal of Musculoskeletal & Neuronal Interaction.* 7;344–345.

Tinetti, MC, Inouye, SK, Gill, TM, et al. (1995). Shared Risk Factors for Falls, Incontinence, and Functional Dependence. Unifying the Approach to Geriatric Syndromes. *Journal of the American Medical Association.* 273(17);1348–1353.

*U.S. Department of Health and Human Services.* (2008). *Physical Activity Guidelines for Americans.* Washington, DC [Online]. https://health.gov/dietaryguidelines/2015/guidelines/appendix-1/

*World Health Organization.* (2013). *Diet and Physical Activity Factsheet. Secondary Diet and Physical Activity Factsheet* [Online]. www.who.int/dietphysicalactivity/fact_sheet_in activity/en/index. html

# PART III

# Exercise Comes of Age

# 7
# THE RATIONALE FOR GERIATRIC EXERCISE

As an older adult, John was aware that he was having some difficulties working in the yard. Last week, in particular, while cutting the grass, his legs were hurting and he was physically exhausted. He knew something was not right, so he stopped without finishing the yard. He wondered if it was his age and the fact that he was overweight and living a sedentary lifestyle. Then, it became apparent to John that the muscle fatigue and joint pain meant that he needed to buy a riding lawn mower. Having crossed the conscious threshold of being young and strong to old and weak begs the question, "Why didn't John think about starting a walking program to correct for the age-related changes in the muscles?" Surely, lifting weights would have helped to increase the size, strength, and endurance of his muscles.

Aging is a composition of subtle physiological and musculoskeletal changes that set the stage for progressive weakness and/or disability. Lifestyle factors do matter, but actually they are seldom discussed among friends much less with healthcare providers. Also, interestingly, lifestyle factors undergo changes with new research just when everything seems to be going great. The threshold for change usually takes place when a significant weakness, impairment, and/or dysfunction becomes apparent, such as when a sedentary individual experiences difficulty trying to do something that was otherwise easy to do. In the absence of pathology, such transitions are due to age-related changes in key organ systems.

---

### BOX 7.1  IMPORTANT CONSEQUENCES OF AGE-RELATED CHANGES.

Aging impairs exercise capacity by increasing the physiological effort (as indicated by heart rate, blood pressure, and respiration) to perform the same work (such as brisk walking) that was easier 10 or 20 years ago (Singh 2002). As a result, the older adult tends to avoid the activity that often leads to increased sedentariness (Grembowski et al. 1993).

DOI: 10.4324/9781003119920-10

—Singh, MAF. (2002). Exercise Comes of Age: Rationale and Recommendations for a Geriatric Exercise Prescription. *Journal of Gerontology: Medical Sciences.* 57(5);262–282.

—Grembowski, D, Patrick, D, Diehr, P, et al. (1993). Self-Efficacy and Health Behavior Among Older Adults. *Journal of Health and Social Behavior.* 34;89–104.

## Benefits of Exercise for Aging Adults

The chronic adaptations to aerobic training allow for the opportunity to exercise without the limitations typically associated with a sedentary lifestyle and aging. For example, an increase in cardiorespiratory fitness (as measured by the subject's maximal oxygen consumption, $VO_2$ max) has a strong inverse association with the risk of coronary artery disease (CAD). The higher the $VO_2$ max, the lower the risk of CAD. The primary inroad to understanding the association between the two is related to the decrease in serum low-density lipoprotein (LDL) cholesterol with aerobic exercise while also increasing high-density lipoprotein (HDL) cholesterol. These benefits of exercise result in a lower risk of heart disease (Boone 2014).

Type II muscle fibers (also referred to as fast-twitch muscle fibers) are used in powerful, quick movements (Lexell 1995) like sprinting. Loss of fast-twitch fibers leads to disability and frailty that is associated with increased illness and mortality with aging. Resistance training increases muscle mass and strength regardless of the age of a person (Roubenoff 2000). The benefits of resistance training also include improvements in the elderly adult's balance, gait stability, sleep quality, mental health, immune system, and overall cognitive and physical functioning (Mernitz & Mcdermott 2004). These exercise benefits make life easier and safer with the age-related changes.

Although the biological changes of aging impair physiological well-being and functional capacity, the cardiovascular and musculoskeletal adaptations to regular aerobic exercise and resistance training help to overcome the physical limitations. Both types of exercises produce specific benefits that have been shown to reverse the changes associated with aging. Otherwise, without overloading the muscles with resistance training exercises while also continuing to avoid aerobic exercise, the lack of exercise-augmented adaptations allows the aging process to result in visible changes recognized as frailty.

---

**BOX 7.2  OLD AGE, LOSS OF MUSCLE MASS, AND RESISTANCE TRAINING.**

The integrity of musculoskeletal function is defined by the overall performance of the muscular system, which is impacted by aging and exacerbated by physical inactivity and/or sedentariness. Apart from the obvious physiological benefits of aerobic exercise on heart rate, blood pressure, and other cardiorespiratory responses, musculoskeletal integrity is defined largely by the size of the muscle mass that is responsible for a movement pattern. Hence, strength, power, and muscle endurance are dictated largely by muscle size, which can be maintained or increased by resistance training while aging.

Conversely, the positive side of engaging in regular exercise is its link to better mind and body health and function. It isn't that difficult to grasp the negative feelings that aging adults must deal with when they look at the decrease in the size of their arm muscles. What was an impressive biceps brachii is now a thin and weak muscle that is either unable to lift objects that were easy to lift years earlier or does so with discomfort and/or pain. This is true for most aging adults who lose 20% to 40% of their muscle mass with aging (Frontera et al. 1991; Hughes et al. 2002). Ultimately, the decrease in aerobic activities and the failure to overload the muscles with resistance training along with the physiological and musculoskeletal changes of aging and disuse renders older and elderly men and women weak and frail.

While frailty is the outcome of both aging and a sedentary lifestyle, it is possible to age without becoming frail and weak. Fortunately, the benefits of regular exercise (i.e., exercise medicine) are the physiological changes of aging that are modifiable by aerobic and resistance training programs. As pointed out by Singh (2002), several of these changes are presented in the following categories: (a) exercise and work capacity; (b) cardiorespiratory function; (c) nutritional status; and (d) metabolic considerations.

---

### BOX 7.3 AGE-RELATED CHANGES THAT RESULT FROM REGULAR EXERCISE.

| Exercise and Work Capacity | Aging and Disuse Effect | Exercise Effect |
|---|---|---|
| Aerobic capacity (VO$_2$ max) | Decrease | Increase |
| Submaximal exercise HR and BP | Increase | Decrease |
| Muscle strength and endurance | Decrease | Increase |
| Oxidative enzyme capacity | Decrease | Increase |
| **Cardiorespiratory Function** | Decrease | Increase |
| Stroke volume | Decrease | Increase |
| Cardiac output | Decrease | Increase |
| Skeletal muscle blood flow | Decrease | Increase |
| Capillary distensibility | Decrease | Increase |
| Tidal volume | Decrease | Increase |
| **Nutritional** | Decrease | Increase |
| Total energy expenditure | Decrease | Increase |
| Total body potassium and calcium | Decrease | Increase |
| Protein synthesis rate/turnover | Decrease | Increase |
| **Metabolic** | Increase | Decrease |
| Glycogen storage capacity | Increase | Decrease or no change |
| Glycogen synthase | Decrease or no change | Increase or no change |
| SNS response to stress | | |
| LDL cholesterol | | |
| HDL cholesterol | | |

A higher level of aerobic capacity is linked to the exercise increase in physical fitness that decreases the elderly adults' disability and mortality. Also, the icing on the cake is that resistance training combats myopathy and osteopenia while increasing muscle strength, endurance, and function. Additional benefits of both types of exercise are the increase in bone health and postural stability. But, unfortunately, only 30 out of every 100 adults 65 years of age and older engage in regular exercise (Mernitz & McDermott 2004). This is a major healthcare problem since physical inactivity is associated with a greater burden of chronic diseases and decreased functional status.

A by-product of a restricted aerobic exercise is an increase in the load placed on the cardiovascular system. For example, the increase in heart rate (HR) and systolic blood pressure (SBP) is a common hemodynamic response to being physically inactive, which increases the work of the heart. This point is illustrated in the calculation of myocardial oxygen consumption [$MVO_2 = .14 (HR \times SBP \times .01) - 6.3$], while at rest and when engaged in a brisk walk (Boone 2014):

$$MVO_2 = .14 (HR \times SBP \times .01) - 6.3$$
$$= .14 (70 \times 120 \times .01) - 6.3$$
$$= 5.46 \text{ mL·}100 \text{ g LV·min}^{-1} \text{ (at rest, a physically active person)}$$

$$MVO_2 = .14 (HR \times SBP \times .01) - 6.3$$
$$= .14 (85 \times 130 \times .01) - 6.3$$
$$= 9.17 \text{ mL·}100 \text{ g LV·min}^{-1} \text{ (at rest, physically inactive person)}$$

$$MVO_2 = .14 (HR \times SBP \times .01) - 6.3$$
$$= .14 (110 \times 130 \times .01) - 6.3$$
$$= 13.72 \text{ mL·}100 \text{ g LV·min}^{-1} \text{ (brisk walk, physically active)}$$

$$MVO_2 = .14 (HR \times SBP \times .01) - 6.3$$
$$= .14 (140 \times 150 \times .01) - 6.3$$
$$= 23.10 \text{ mL·}100 \text{ g LV·min}^{-1} \text{ (brisk walk, physically inactive)}$$

Note that being physically inactive increases the work of the heart, as indicated in the calculation of $MVO_2$. At rest, it is 9.17 mL·100 g LV·min$^{-1}$ when physically inactive. But, with aerobic training (such as when engaging in a daily brisk walk), the resting HR and SBP are lower than the person who is physically inactive. Both physiological variables represent what is called double product (or rate pressure product). Thus, the products of HR and SBP are primarily responsible for the work of the heart that is reflected in the increase in stroke volume (SV), which is the volume of blood ejected from the ventricles to the body. The volume that is ejected from the left ventricle is full of oxygen that is delivered to the skeletal muscles to provide for the contraction of muscles so that movement is possible.

The good news is that older adults can start slowly and benefit from regular exercise. The payoff is in better health. It is common knowledge that exercise helps the frail person feel better while also preventing and/or controlling many chronic diseases. After all, isn't exercise known to stop or prevent the deterioration of the body by helping to control weight and prevent obesity, lower the risk of heart disease by decreasing high cholesterol and blood pressure, lower blood sugar level to help decrease the risk of type 2 diabetes, slow the decrease in bone density with aging, and reduce the risk of falling (Boone 2014).

---

### BOX 7.4 THE IMPORTANCE OF REGULAR EXERCISE.

As Box 7.3 indicates, regular exercise administered by ASEP Board-Certified Exercise Physiologists results in positive effects that attenuate loss of strength and power with aging while also reversing the frailty phenotype and decreasing functional deficits of frail adults. Hence, older adults will remain physically independent for a longer period of their life.

---

Exercise physiologists are aware that regular exercise helps adults of all ages to feel better. Their research has demonstrated many times that physical activity has a favorable influence on the mind and body. Unfortunately, for decades no one (including physicians) took the research findings seriously.

## Staying Active and Aging

Today, talking about staying active and prescribing exercise as medicine are topics of considerable interest. Most healthcare professionals believe that exercise is the key to keeping the mind as well as the body healthy and strong. Of particular interest is the decrease in ischemic heart disease and the increased integrity of the musculoskeletal system. Exercise physiologists, in particular, are keenly aware of the importance of staying active throughout life, especially with aging. Regular exercise helps to improve and/or maintain cardiovascular endurance, muscle strength, and flexibility. The most common method of determining the influence of regular exercise on the body is to measure a person's oxygen uptake ($VO_2$). The units for reporting $VO_2$ are liters per minute ($L \cdot min^{-1}$), which is an absolute number or milliliters per kilogram of bodyweight per minute ($mL \cdot kg^{-1} \cdot min^{-1}$), which is a relative number. The latter unit allows for the comparison of maximum oxygen uptake ($VO_2$ max, also known as functional aerobic capacity) of individuals with different body sizes.

As you would expect, the $VO_2$ max of a physically inactive aging adult isn't very high. While their respiratory system is responsible for bringing in the maximum amount of oxygen from the atmosphere, the blood between the right ventricle and the left atrium (i.e., the pulmonary circuit) transports the oxygen in combination with hemoglobin ($HbO_2$) to the heart where it is pumped from the left ventricle throughout the circulatory system to the muscles. Oxygen uptake and carbon dioxide output ($VCO_2$) at the cellular level are measured during the respiratory gas exchange. The $O_2$ consumed during the cellular metabolism is equal to $VO_2$. The increase in metabolism during exercise is reflective of the increased need for $O_2$ consumed by the electron transport system (ETS) in the mitochondria to produce adenosine triphosphate (ATP). The ATP is the energy used to produce muscle contraction. Thus, exercise increases the work and efficiency of the heart, lungs, and muscles that in return provides for movement and quality of life.

By age 75, most adults are not physically active. As a result, over half of the functional capacity of the cardiorespiratory system (i.e., physical fitness) has been lost. The decrease in fitness compromises the function of the heart, which results in a decrease in independence and quality of life due to the decrease in left ventricular function. As a result, there is a decrease in cardiac output (Q), which is the product of heart rate (HR) and stroke volume (SV). Even though the arterial blood is essentially full of $O_2$, the decrease in SV and, therefore, the decrease in Q is primarily the reason for the aging adult's decrease in $VO_2$ and physical ability to exercise. Also, the low cardiorespiratory fitness has been shown to be a strong and independent predictor of mortality risk (Wei et al. 1999).

Not only are physical fitness and regular exercise excellent means of aging well but also both allow for an assessment of physiological function on cardiovascular morbidity and mortality rates. Therefore, by demonstrating that $VO_2$ is increased after an exercise program (given that $VO_2$ = ATP, which = Energy, which = Muscle Contraction, then exercise = Life), statistically speaking, there should be a decrease in cardiovascular mortality (i.e., $VO_2$ = Life). This is especially the case when the exercise program results in the expenditure of more than 2000 $kcal \cdot wk^{-1}$ versus 500 $kcal \cdot wk^{-1}$ (Paffenbarger et al. 1986). While it should not be surprising that regular exercise (a form of physical activity) is inversely related to the risk of developing heart disease and stroke (Manson et al. 1995), it is still not a popular alternative to taking a pill by the majority of the population in the United States and worldwide (Box 7.5).

---

### BOX 7.5   WHY DO WE SUFFER?

Jean Mayer said, "For we in this generation and in the United States are the pampered of our planet. We are the fat of the land: never in history, nowhere else in the world have such numbers of human beings eaten so much, exerted themselves so little, and become and remained so fat. We have come suddenly into the land of milk and honey, and we look it. And we suffer because of it."

---

## Exercise Medicine

Exercise is the recommended treatment for hypertension, type 2 diabetes, obesity, elevated lipids, thrombosis, and coronary artery disease just as prescription drugs are recognized as medical treatment for the same diseases and/or conditions. This means exercise is the equivalent of a drug prescribed by a physician and thus should be thought of as medicine. For decades, there have been numerous reports that exercise prevents the development of high blood pressure (Paffenbarger et al. 1983), increases the sensitivity to insulin while decreasing glucose production by the liver (Wasserman & Zinman 1995), decreases low-density lipoprotein (LDL) cholesterol (Wood et al. 1991), decreases blood platelet aggregation (Stratton et al. 1991), and increases the activity of the parasympathetic nervous system with a resulting decrease in double product (DP) and myocardial oxygen consumption ($MVO_2$).

In non-frail aging adults, positive physiological and musculoskeletal adaptations result from prescribing exercise medicine at low-to-moderate-intensity aerobic exercise that is performed 3 to 5 $times \cdot wk^{-1}$ for ~20 to 60 $min \cdot d^{-1}$. Regular exercise increases the efficiency of the respiratory system. In fact, at a specific workload after aerobic training, expired ventilation ($V_E$) is decreased due to the product of an increase in tidal volume ($V_T$) and a decrease in frequency of breaths ($F_b$). Also, the diaphragm and the external intercostals become more efficient during breathing. This means less oxygen is necessary to do the same amount of work, thus allowing for more oxygen to be used by the muscles.

The oxygen that diffuses from the alveoli into the pulmonary blood is transported by the increase in hemoglobin (Hb) per 100 mL of blood. For comparison, the non-exercise trained Hb is ~15 g·100 mL, while the trained concentration is ~17 g·100 mL of blood. Therefore, with the increase in Hb, the oxygen-carrying capacity of the blood is increased from ~20.1 mL of $O_2$ per 100 mL (i.e., 1.34 mL of $O_2$ × 15 g·100 mL) to ~23 mL·100 mL of blood. This means that the development of energy in the form of ATP in the electron transport system (ETS) of the mitochondria (that requires oxygen) benefits from the increase in oxygen in the blood that ultimately produces more energy for muscle contraction. With aerobic training, there is also an increase in the number of respiratory capillaries with an increase in oxygen diffusion from the lungs into the pulmonary blood that is transported to the left ventricle from which it is pumped into the arterial system. Hence, there is more oxygen to dissociate from the $HbO_2$ to diffuse into the muscle cells to produce more energy.

The left ventricular contraction becomes stronger with regular aerobic exercise. Each ventricular contraction sends blood into the circulatory system, and it does so with a lower HR at rest and during exercise that allows for increased filling of the ventricles. Thus, the increase in ventricular contractility results in a larger volume of blood ejected per beat (SV) with a lower HR. The decrease in $MVO_2$ is directly related to the decrease in HR and systolic blood pressure (SBP). The product of both variables is double product (DP). The lower the DP during exercise (such as a brisk walk), the lesser the oxygen needed by the heart to deliver the blood to the muscles.

Regular exercise increases motor unit activation and transmission of nerve impulses that are responsible for increasing muscle strength and endurance. Thus, overall, the increase in oxygen and ATP produces an increase in muscular activity, which increases $VO_2$ max and elasticity of the arterial system along with a decrease in LDL or "bad" cholesterol. There is also an increase in high-density lipoprotein (HDL) or "good" cholesterol that provides for an increase in protection from coronary artery disease (CAD).

Although low-density lipoprotein (LDL) cholesterol concentration is the primary index of cardiovascular disease risk, Millan et al. (2009) suggest that the total cholesterol-to-HDL ratio is a better marker of the risk of heart disease than LDL cholesterol levels alone. Regular exercise improves the ratio of total cholesterol (CHL) to HDL cholesterol. Ideally, the ratio should be below 4. For example, if the CHL:HDL ratio is 6 or greater, there is a higher risk of heart disease (e.g., 180 mg·dL$^{-1}$ ÷ 30 mg·dL$^{-1}$). This is the case even though the total CHL is less than 200 mg·dL$^{-1}$. In this case, the lower the HDL cholesterol, the higher the risk of CAD. Fortunately, regular exercise increases HDL cholesterol while lowering total CHL (Brown 1996). While cardiac mortality is decreased in aging adults who engage in regular exercise, there is also an improvement in recovery after a cardiac event (Austin et al. 2005; Ning & Chen 2010).

---

### BOX 7.6  LEVELS OF HEALTHY CHOLESTEROL.

Cholesterol in the United States is measured in milligrams per deciliter (mg·dL$^{-1}$). The guidelines for healthy cholesterol levels are as follows: (a) total cholesterol below 170 mg·dL$^{-1}$; (b) LDL cholesterol less than 100 mg·dL$^{-1}$; (c) HDL cholesterol above 45 mg·dL$^{-1}$; and (d) non-HDL cholesterol less than 120 mg·dL$^{-1}$.

Regular exercise helps to bring about the regression of atheroma in major arteries, thus providing protection against CAD. Not only does exercise help decrease the triglyceride levels in the blood but also it increases the loss of body fat, decreases emotional tension and stress, improves psychological health, and is an excellent treatment for mild to moderate depression (Sung 2009; Tanaka 2009). Clearly, exercise is medicine and it should be prescribed by Board-Certified Exercise Physiologists. Older frail subjects should start with 5- to 10-min sessions and slowly increase their duration of exercise. As aging frail adults adapt physically and mentally to the exercise medicine prescription, they will reduce the amount of saturated fat in their diet, lose weight that will help lower their LDL cholesterol, and have more energy.

## Final Thoughts

It is common to recognize aging by changes in posture and walking patterns. It is less common to acknowledge the composition of physiological and musculoskeletal changes that more often than not results in progressive weakness and/or disability in older adults. In particular, the decrease in lean muscle mass and bone density along with the curved and compressed spinal column that contributes to the adult's weakness, fatigue, inflammation, pain, stiffness, and the likelihood of falling and fractures.

---

**BOX 7.7   DESCRIPTION OF AGING SKELETAL MUSCLE MASS.**

Frontera et al. (2000) measured the cross-sectional area of male subjects' thighs 12 years apart to identify changes in lean muscle mass. The subjects were 65.4 ± 4.2 years of age when the first measurement was made, and they were 77.6 ± 4.0 years of age at the second measurement. At the onset of the study, the measurement of the thigh muscles was ~136 cm$^2$. Twelve years later, it was 116 cm$^2$, which was almost a 15% decrease in the subjects' thigh mass. As expected, the decrease in muscle cross-sectional area was linked to a decrease in muscle strength of the knee extensors and flexors.

—Frontera, WR, Hughes, VA, Fielding, RA, et al. (2000). Aging of Skeletal Muscle: A 12-yr Longitudinal Study. *Journal of Applied Physiology*. 88(4);1321–1326.

---

The adaptations to regular aerobic exercise training and resistance training exercises help to overcome the physical and mental limitations associated with aging. In short, the frail person feels better, especially since exercise has come of age as the treatment for many chronic diseases, including hypertension, type 2 diabetes, obesity, elevated lipids, thrombosis, and coronary artery disease just as prescription drugs are recognized as medical treatment for the same diseases and/or conditions.

When exercise is prescribed by an ASEP Board-Certified Exercise Physiologist, it is considered the equivalent of a drug prescribed by a physician and should, therefore, be thought of as medicine (Boone 2012). While the recommendation for exercise is client and/or patient specific, it is generally in the range of 20 to 40 min 3 d·wk$^{-1}$ of aerobic exercise (e.g., a brisk walk or jog) at a light to moderate intensity to produce an improvement in the cardiovascular system. Additionally, given the age-related issues that result from the decrease in lean muscle mass (particularly among women), strength training that includes 1 to 3 sets of 8 to 12 repetitions at 70% of 1 repetition maximum 2 to 3 d·wk⁻¹ is recommended (and adjusted accordingly) for frail adults (Hawkins & Wiswell 2003). Exercise is the medicine to reverse and restore independent functioning in elderly frail adults.

There isn't any question that exercise is the best medicine for frailty. The problem is getting the medical community, physicians, in particular, to work with exercise physiologists in getting their patients to be more physically active to fight the loss of strength and cardiovascular integrity.

Another problem is that most elderly adults do not have the desire to exercise. They will say that they don't have either the equipment or the time to exercise. Down deep they question whether exercise is medicine, and so they would rather take a pill to improve their health.

## References

Austin, J, Williams, R, Ross, I, et al. (2005). Randomized Controlled Trial of Cardiac Rehabilitation in Elderly Patients with Heart Failure. *European Journal of Heart Failure.* 7(3);411–417.

Boone, T. (2012). *Exercise Physiology as a Healthcare Profession.* Lewiston, NY: The Edwin Mellen Press.

Boone, T. (2014). *Introduction to Exercise Physiology.* Burlington, MA: Jones & Bartlett Learning.

Brown, HL. (1996). *Lifetime Fitness.* Scottsdale, AZ: Gorsuch Scarisbrick, Publishers.

Frontera, W, Hughes, V, Lutz, K, Evans, W. (1991). A Cross-Sectional Study of Muscle Strength and Mass in 45- to 78-yr-old Men and Women. *Journal of Applied Physiology.* 71;644–650.

Hawkins, SA, Wiswell, RA. (2003). Rate and Mechanism of Maximal Oxygen Consumption Decline with Aging: Implications for Exercise Training. *Sports Medicine,* 33(12);877–888.

Hughes, V, Frontera, W, Roubenoff, R, et al. (2002). Longitudinal Changes in Body Composition Changes in Older Men and Women: Role of Body Weight Change and Physical Activity. *American Journal of Clinical Nutrition.* 76;473–481.

Lexell, J. (1995). Human Aging, Muscle Mass, and Fiber Type Composition. *Journal of Gerontology: A Biological Science & Medical Science.* 50;11–16.

Manson, JE, Stampfer, MJ, Willett, WC, Colditz, GA, Speizer, FE, Hennekens, CH. (1995). Physical Activity and Incidence of Coronary Heart Disease and Stroke in Women. *Circulation.* 9;927.

Mernitz, H, McDermott, AY. (2004). Exercise and the Elderly: A Scientific Rational for Exercise Prescription. *JCOM.* 11(2);106–116.

Millan, J, Pinto, X, Munoz, A, et al. (2009). Lipoprotein Ratios: Physiological Significance and Clinical Usefulness in Cardiovascular Prevention. *Vascular Health and Risk Management.* 5;757–765.

Ning, C, Chen, W. (2010). Summaries of Nursing Care-Related Systematic Reviews from the Cochrane Library: Exercise-Based Rehabilitation for Coronary Heart Disease. *The Journal of Cardiovascular Nursing.* 25(5);379–380.

Paffenbarger, RS, Hyde, RT, Wing, A, et al. (1986). Physical Activity, All-Cause Mortality, and Longevity of College Alumni. *New England Journal of Medicine.* 314;605–613.

Paffenbarger, RS, Wing, AL, Hyde, RD. (1983). Physical Activity and Incidence of Hypertension in College Alumni. *American Journal of Epidemiology.* 117;245–257.

Roubenoff, R. (2000). Sarcopenia and Its Implications for the Elderly. *European Journal of Clinical Nutrition.* 54(3);40–47.

Singh, MAF. (2002). Exercise Comes of Age: Rationale and Recommendations for a Geriatric Exercise Prescription. *Journal of Gerontology: Medical Sciences.* 57(5);262–282.

Stratton, JR, Chandler, WL, Schwartz, RS, et al. (1991). Effects of Physical Conditioning on Fibrinolytic Variables in Young and Old Healthy Adults. *Circulation.* 83;1692–1697.

Sung, K. (2009). The Effect of 16-week Group Exercise Program on Physical Function and Mental Health of Elderly Korean Women in Long-Term Assisted Living Facility. *Journal of Cardiovascular Nursing,* 24(5);344–351.

Tanaka, H. (2009). Habitual Exercise for the Elderly. *Family Community Health*. 32(1);57–65.

Wasserman, DH, Zinman, B. (1995). In: Ruderman, N, Devlin, JT. (Editors), *The Health Professional's Guide to Diabetes and Exercise*. Alexandria, VA: American Diabetes Association, 29–47.

Wei, M, Kampert, JB, Barlow, CE, et al. (1999). Relationship Between Low Cardiorespiratory Fitness and Mortality in Normal-Weight, Overweight, and Obese Men. *Journal of the American Medical Association*. 282;1547–1553.

Wood, PD, Stefanick, ML, Williams, PT, Haskell, WL. (1991). The Effects on Plasma Lipoproteins of a Prudent Weight-Reducing Diet, With or Without Exercise in Overweight Men and Women. *New England Journal of Medicine*. 325;919–924.

# 8
# THE CHALLENGE OF IMPLEMENTING EXERCISE MEDICINE

There are three major challenges that must be better understood, evaluated, and engaged to increase and support the use of exercise medicine by the ASEP Board-Certified Exercise Physiologists: (1) aging and choices, (2) the medical profession and the use of prescription drugs, and (3) the conditions of society that do not support an active exercise lifestyle. These challenges are real and whether they function singularly or together in a different arrangement, it is difficult to break with status quo and embrace new thinking and new healthcare possibilities.

## Aging and Choices

The expectation of living longer in America is increasing even though many adults do not stick to a regular exercise schedule. Yet it is clear that going for several short walks throughout the day is better than not walking at all. This point is especially important for the fastest-growing segment of the population, which is the 85-and-older age group. Despite being 85 years old, many elderly adults have chronic and progressive diseases. Naturally, it is better to be 85 years old without one or more chronic diseases or a disability that requires assistance with many of the daily activities.

Fortunately, it is possible for more adults to achieve old age without an illness like congestive heart failure or high blood pressure. Regular exercise can help delay or completely avoid dozens of different chronic diseases. But aging adults must engage in regular exercise while also making choices to live a healthier life as they age.

---

**BOX 8.1  STEPS TO SUCCESSFUL AGING.**

Drive less, walk more. Avoid cigarette smoking. Strengthen the muscles. Laugh more, have fun. Focus on eating a healthy diet. Set realistic goals. Develop friendships. Forget about competition. Take the stairs. Be nice to others. Accept change. Moderate alcohol. Follow your passions.

---

DOI: 10.4324/9781003119920-11

Although regular exercise primarily is thought of as aerobic exercise, it is important to engage in all four types of exercise: endurance, strength, balance, and flexibility. Each one has its own benefits. Also, doing one kind often improves the aging adults' ability to do the others. For example, aerobic exercise doesn't have to be just walking or jogging. It can be swimming, biking, dancing, and playing basketball or tennis. It can also be yard work such as raking or mowing. Physical inactivity, regardless of age, can be significantly reduced with the guidance of an ASEP Board-Certified Exercise Physiologist who understands that exercise medicine is medical treatment (Boone 2009).

Although aging is a multifactorial process that involves changes associated with normal aging, the effects of lifestyle and genetics add to the decrease in the cardiorespiratory and muscular systems (Boone 2014). For these reasons, it is clear that aging and frail patients need professional supervision to help with living an active and fit lifestyle. For this reason, every aging adult should be asked about exercise at every visit to a physician's office and, when needed, provided with an exercise prescription by an ASEP exercise physiologist (Boone 2007). Exercise medicine is a powerful prescription for the prevention and treatment of chronic diseases, for decreasing the harmful effects of obesity, and for lowering mortality rates and disabilities. But it is important to remember that it must be implemented by a profession-specific healthcare professional, which is the ASEP Board-Certified Exercise Physiologist (ASEP 2019).

## The Medical Profession and the Use of Prescription Drugs

How can the medical profession improve the health of their patients without modifying their behavior regarding exercise, smoking, and diet if they don't refer them to qualified healthcare professionals? The evidence indicates that they cannot and, therefore, their patients suffer the consequences. For example, patients who smoke should be referred to a smoking cessation program. Patients who are overweight or obese should be referred to a dietitian, and patients who are physically inactive and/or need help to safely engage in regular exercise should be referred to a qualified exercise physiologist (who should be recognized by the medical profession as an integral part of the healthcare team).

---

**BOX 8.2   THE ASEP PERSPECTIVE REGARDING CERTIFICATION.**

The **ASEP Board of Certification** declares that the professional Exercise Physiologist requires certification according to the ASEP certification procedures, and that the health and welfare of the public is protected by Exercise Physiologists who are academically qualified and certified as EPCs to practice exercise physiology.

---

But, despite the benefits of exercise, very few physicians provide their patients with an exercise prescription much less refer them to an ASEP exercise physiologist. In fact, most physicians appear unaware of the fact that ASEP is the professional organization of exercise physiologists (Boone 2001). Physicians no longer have to be prepared to counsel and prescribe exercise to patients. After all, given the number of patients per day, their lack of time and remuneration, as well as their lack of experience in prescribing exercise medicine is well-known. There is no secret that incorporating exercise medicine into the medical curriculum would help physicians understand the value and importance of working with ASEP exercise physiologists.

---

### BOX 8.3   ASEP DEFINITIONS.

**Exercise Physiologist** means a person who has an academic degree in exercise physiology, who is certified by ASEP to practice exercise physiology (as an EPC, i.e., Board-Certified Exercise Physiologist), or who has a doctorate degree with an academic degree or emphasis in exercise physiology from an accredited college or university.

**Exercise Physiology** means the identification of physiological mechanisms underlying physical activity, the comprehensive delivery of treatment services concerned with the analysis, improvement, and maintenance of health and fitness, rehabilitation of heart disease and other chronic diseases and/or disabilities, and the professional guidance and counsel of athletes and others interested in athletics, sports training, and human adaptability to acute and chronic exercise.

---

The problem is that it is easier to prescribe drugs than to target and discuss physical inactivity as a key risk factor for chronic diseases. Fortunately, with the existence of ASEP, physicians can counsel and encourage their patients to seek the help and guidance of ASEP exercise physiologists with training in exercise medicine and prescribing exercise to their clients and/or patients.

The ASEP leaders are doing what they can to increase public awareness about the health concerns that result from physical inactivity and, where the opportunity arises, counseling inactive aging adults (and frail adults) to start an exercise program. They are concerned that patients are not being told about the importance of exercise as a standard of care for all adults to prevent or treat frailty. They want to know why physicians consider fitness as something altogether different from health care. This is a major problem, given the health hazards associated with a sedentary lifestyle. Why is bariatric surgery paid for by insurance companies, but the help of an exercise physiologist to implement an exercise prescription to decrease excess body fat is paid by the client?

It should be obvious that these are serious concerns. Most research regarding the health benefits of exercise agrees that the majority of the teenagers, adults, and aging frail individuals are on the wrong path. The solution is not more medical drugs. As a society, we have to look to the power within ourselves to become more responsible for our health and well-being.

The medical community should start collaborating with qualified exercise physiologists as the healthcare professionals of the 21st century. The health and sickness crisis of adults becoming frail as they age will not just go away. The question of considerable importance is this: "Will the medical community reach out to the ASEP exercise physiologists?" After all, the future of each adult is more important than the present way of dealing with health issues.

## Society's Failure to Live an Active Lifestyle

Based on the information presented earlier, prescribing exercise isn't as easy or as common as you might think it should be. There are several challenges that must be dealt with. Aside from the organizational differences and concerns, there are existing educational issues that influence different professions and their duty to the public. Third, aside from exercise as the long-sought-after drug to extend life by preventing chronic disease and frailty, why is it that society prefers a pill in a bottle and not in the form of actual exercise? Why has society neglected exercise as a standard treatment for a life free from chronic disease and/or disability?

The answer to the last question is complex. No doubt part of the answer is that most people are more interested in nice clothes, a big house, several cars, and being successful (i.e., a big salary) at work than doing what is necessary to maintain one's health and fitness. It goes without saying that financial success is at the top of the list. Therefore, it is easier for the majority of the physicians to prescribe a drug to decrease blood pressure or cholesterol than to talk with a patient about the amazing benefits of exercise medicine. They know the patient isn't interested and the medical community isn't prepared to fulfill his or her needs. The lack of interest in exercising is in many ways the equivalent of living on borrowed time. The forces of physical inactivity work to reduce the body to a frail condition with diminished freedom accompanied by an abundance of mental and physical health problems.

The folly of the masses is neglecting the importance of exercise medicine. There is no reward for remaining ignorant to the false beliefs and assumptions that exercise is something children do. Such thinking is a complete meltdown in mental power that can improve one's health. That is why it is critical that ASEP Board-Certified Exercise Physiologists are recognized as the means to stop with the pills and start the process of moving from disease and disability to a healthier lifestyle. But, as long as physicians continue to avoid their professional and legal responsibility for promoting exercise medicine to their patients, it is unlikely there will be a decrease in non-communicable diseases, obesity, and mortality rates that are linked to a lifestyle of physical inactivity.

Society's problem is mind–body paralysis. Without transformation from one of inactivity to an active lifestyle, the good news of the effects of exercise medicine will be very slow to materialize. The evidence is clear that we need a true cure to our physical inactivity, which is exercise medicine. Exercise is a very powerful medicine to treat and prevent mind and body diseases, to avoid the effects of obesity, and to decrease frailty. The momentous question before us is, "How can we reshape our way of living to fit and conform to a healthier lifestyle with an increase in functional capacity and quality of life?"

The American health dilemma is laziness. The present state of countries around the world makes exercise medicine the only means to surviving the greatest public health problem of our time. For this reason, physicians have a responsibility to refer their inactive patients before they become obese, sick, or frail to an ASEP exercise physiologist to provide both a cardiovascular and a musculoskeletal assessment followed by a personalized exercise prescription for better health and well-being.

---

### BOX 8.4 LAZINESS IS KILLING US.

Two thousand years ago, Hippocrates, the Father of Modern Medicine, hit the nail on the head when he said, that if we all had "the right amount of nourishment and exercise, not too little and not too much, we would have found the safest way to health." Bingo.

## Final Thoughts

It is clear to the ASEP leadership that the intersection of regular exercise as medicine for better health falls closest to the profession of exercise physiology. For this reason, it makes sense that ASEP Board-Certified Exercise Physiologists should lead the effort in promoting regular exercise among clients and patients (Boone 2016). Exercise physiologists have the academic training in both the classroom and the laboratory in understanding the physiology of exercise to help anyone interested in beginning, maintaining, or increasing physiological performance. It is also clear that these ASEP healthcare professionals can have their greatest impact on society's health by promoting and monitoring the medical benefits of regular exercise. In addition, physicians should consider exercise as an essential part of the treatment for all patients to stay healthy. An important job for exercise physiologists is to help sedentary older people to participate in regular physical exercise to increase life expectancy. Exercise must become a habit and not an option, especially since the risk of mortality for men with a cardiopulmonary capacity equal to or greater than 10 metabolic equivalents (METs) is three times lower than in men with a cardiorespiratory fitness of less than or equal to four METs (Kokkinos & Myers 2010). Similarly, according to Blair et al. 1989, the same has been observed in women with a cardiorespiratory fitness greater than or equal to nine METs compared to women with a cardiorespiratory fitness of less than or equal to six METs.

Also, just as patients starting an exercise program should understand there is no amount of exercise that does not have an impact on their cardiorespiratory fitness and health, organizational leadership should take every opportunity to engage in positive discussions regarding "the importance of working together on behalf of society's physical and mental well-being" and "the necessity of demonstrating respect for philosophic differences due to professional goals and objectives."

## References

*American Society of Exercise Physiologists*. (2019). *The Organization* [Online]. www.asep.org/organization/

Blair, SN, Kohl, HW III, Paffenbarger, RS Jr, et al. (1989). Physical Fitness and All-Cause Mortality. A Prospective Study of Healthy Men and Women. *Journal of the American Medical Association*, 262(17);2395–2401.

Boone, T. (2001). *Professional Development of Exercise Physiology*. Lewiston, NY: The Edwin Mellen Press.

Boone, T. (2007). *Ethical Standards and Professional Credentials*. Lewiston, NY: The Edwin Mellen Press.

Boone, T. (2009). *The Professionalization of Exercise Physiology: Certification, Accreditation, and Standards of Practice of the American Society of Exercise Physiologists (ASEP)*. Lewiston, NY: The Edwin Mellen Press.

Boone, T. (2014). *Introduction to Exercise Physiology*. Burlington, MA: Jones & Bartlett Learning.

Boone, T. (2016). *ASEP's Exercise Medicine Text for Exercise Physiologists*. Sharjah, UAE: Bentham Science Publishers.

Kokkinos, P, Myers, J. (2010). Exercise and Physical Activity: Clinical Outcomes and Applications. *Circulation*. 122(16);1637–1648.

# 9

# RESISTANCE TRAINING AND FRAIL ADULTS

Morbidity and mortality are related to the ability of a muscle group (such as the shoulder flexors) to develop force (i.e., strength) against a resistance and to do so quickly (i.e., power). In a meta-analysis by Cooper et al. (2010), their findings indicate that the risk of death independent of age, sex, and body mass index was increased in adults within the lower handgrip strength quartile. It is clear that grip strength is a strong predictor of subsequent mortality in the older community-dwelling populations.

The loss of muscle mass with aging is known as sarcopenia, which is linked to the decrease in muscular strength, power, and endurance, bone mineral density, exercise tolerance, and the capacity to perform daily activities. For these reasons, the majority of the aging frail adults avoid physical activities due to their difficulty in performing them. The problem is that by avoiding the physical activities they increase the negative effects on their muscular strength and power. For example, regarding the latter, there is an increase in heart rate, blood pressure, frequency of breathing, and tidal volume that indicates a decrease in their cardiorespiratory capacity to handle the associated increase in muscular stress.

However important such training is for other physiological and health reasons, it is important to understand that the problems associated with sarcopenia are not corrected by cardiorespiratory (i.e., aerobic) training. The muscular system requires resistance training exercises to maintain or to increase muscle fiber cross-sectional area and bone density in elderly subjects and aging frail adults with musculoskeletal limitations.

## Effects of Aging and Physical Inactivity

Regardless of the aging adults' typical lack of lifting heavy objects, muscular strength and power are important, and yet they experience declines with aging. Whether it is moving a big chair from one side of a room to the other side, lifting the trash bag out of the trash can, moving the recently purchased food from the car to the kitchen, or getting the luggage in and out of the car, muscle strength is necessary. While other factors may cause problems, such as a low back muscle strain, the failure to maintain the integrity of the muscles throughout the body is likely to create a decrease in movement efficiency as well as the likelihood of an injury from a fall.

DOI: 10.4324/9781003119920-12

---

### BOX 9.1  MUSCULAR STRENGTH DECLINES WITH AGING.

According to Goodpaster et al. (2006), strength declines by 10% to 15% per decade up to the age of 70 years, when the loss accelerates to 25% to 40% per decade. It is possible that this is due to the decreased contribution from the progressively smaller numbers of large tension-producing type II fibers (Frontera et al. 1988; Hughes et al. 2001).

---

Kirkendall and Garrett (1998) also indicate that the muscle mass of the elderly is smaller and weaker because of the loss of type II muscle fibers, which is a problem because fewer type II fibers are associated with a decrease in functional performance. The medicine of choice is resistance training. Although resistance training and/or aerobic training cannot stop the biological aging process, regular exercise can minimize the physiological effects of a sedentary lifestyle while limiting the development of chronic diseases and disabilities. Also, resistance exercises increase bone mass and improve body composition when compared to sedentary older adults.

Ideally, the exercise medicine prescription for older adults and elderly frail adults should include aerobic exercise to improve cardiorespiratory fitness, muscle-strengthening exercises to prevent muscle wasting, osteoporosis, falls, fractures, and a reduction in quality of life, and flexibility exercises to minimize the stress placed on specific muscles and joints (Chodzko-Zajko et al. 2009). This means the ASEP Board-Certified Exercise Physiologist must develop a comprehensive prescription that will address each of the three major areas: (a) aerobic exercise training, (b) muscle-strengthening exercises, and (c) range of motion exercises.

Knowledge of anatomy provides the understanding that muscle-strengthening exercises do not need to be different from one adult to the next in spite of the popularity of gender-specific weight lifting exercises. An individualized approach to training the musculoskeletal system is only necessary for special cases where a musculoskeletal deficiency or injury limits the aging adult's ability to function. Otherwise, all major muscle groups (deltoids, biceps brachii, triceps, hamstrings, quadriceps, gastrocnemius, and soleus) should be exercised to avoid sarcopenia, which results in less protection and more medical cost to deal with the cartilage of the joints. Also, as the age-related neurological changes make the execution of muscular activities less efficient, there is an increase in the fat content of the muscles with a decrease in metabolism. The collective effect results in weakness, an overall decrease in movement, and possibly an increase in disability (Duren et al. 2008).

---

### BOX 9.2  THE COST OF SARCOPENIA.

"As little as a 10% reduction in the prevalence of sarcopenia has the potential to save $1.1 billion in US health care costs."

—Janssen, I, Shepard, DS, Katzmarzyk, PT, Roubenoff, R. (2004). The Health Care Costs of Sarcopenia in the United States. *Journal of Gerontology.* 52;80–85.

---

Just as a low level of aerobic capacity is a strong predictor of an adult's quality of life, mobility, and functional independence, the age-associated decrease in lean muscle mass presents a major challenge for cardiovascular patients to successfully undergo surgery and other medical interventions (Paneni et al. 2017). Fortunately, many of the negative physical and mental effects of aging can be prevented or delayed by engaging in a resistance training program to improve the aging adult's balance, strength, power, coordination, flexibility, and endurance. There are also positive effects of having more energy and endurance, feeling less stressed out, being more independent, and healthier.

Although regular exercise is critical to slowing (and possibly reversing) the severe losses of muscle and bone mass, it is important for elders, near-frail adults, and frail older adults to have a complete physical checkup before starting an exercise program. Following a checkup, it is important to always start slow, follow the physician's advice, and adhere to the exercise recommendations from the Board-Certified Exercise Physiologist. Become comfortable with the movements of one exercise before going on more advanced exercises. Work hard but never overdo it and avoid all ballistic movements, work to execute good form, no breath holding, and increase the weight progressively to maintain relative intensity. In time, the body will respond with better muscular fitness, health, and fewer functional limitations (such as gait velocity, rising from a chair, and stair-climbing power).

## A Resistance Training Guide for Frail Adults

### Part 1: Warm-Up

Resistance training should take place at least 2 d·wk$^{-1}$ (e.g., Tuesday and Thursday). There should be a day of rest between the workouts. Although the list of resistance exercises may vary from one adult to the next, given each person's chronic health conditions, fitness level, and function, the following warm-up is recommended prior to engaging in the resistance exercises for older frail adults.

**First**, walk for 5 min to warm-up the muscles prior to strength training. Walking is an excellent exercise to help direct blood flow to the muscles to get the body ready for the resistance exercises. **Second**, while standing with the arms straight and positioned in front of the shoulders, slowly flex the hips and knees. The upper body should remain erect to assume a semi-squat position. The thighs should be just above horizontal to the floor with the feet fully on the floor. The head and upper body should remain upright while the hips are flexed. The exercise should be performed 8 to 12 times, rest for 1 min, and repeat the exercise to complete 2 sets.

The **third** warm-up exercise requires finding a wall to stand a little farther than arms' length from it. While facing the wall, lean forward to place the hands against the wall at shoulder height and shoulder-width apart. Allow the elbows to flex (i.e., bend) so that the upper body moves toward the wall in a slow, controlled motion. Then, very slowly push back until the arms are straight (Box 9.4A). Repeat the wall push-up 8 to 12 times for 1 set. Rest for 1 min and do a second set. The **fourth** warm-up exercise strengthens the muscles of the forearm that flex the fingers and thumb. These muscles allow for a strong grip. Using a tennis ball or a similar type of ball, squeeze it for 3 to 5 sec. Release the squeeze, take a short rest of 10 to 15 sec, and then repeat the exercise 4 more times. Switch hands and repeat the same steps.

## Part 2: Lifting Weights

After the warm-up, it is time to engage in low- to moderate-intensity resistance training to strengthen the biceps brachii and brachialis muscles (i.e., the primary elbow flexors). The first exercise is the **Biceps Curl** using a 2- to 3-lb dumbbell that can be curled 8 to 10 times. Start with using light weights that will reduce the risk of injury. To begin, stand with a dumbbell in either hand. The feet should be shoulder-width apart with the arm hanging by the side of the thigh with the palm facing forward. Inhale as the weight is slowly raised. Keep the upper arm and elbow close to the side of the body.

Hold the weight at the shoulder for a brief pause. Then, breathe out as the weight is lowered to the starting position. Keep the wrist straight while completing 1 set of 8 to 10 repetitions. After resting for 1 min, complete a second set and then repeat the exercise with the other arm.

The second exercise is the **Overhead Press** to strengthen: (a) the shoulder flexors (i.e., the anterior and middle deltoids, the short and long heads of the biceps brachii at the shoulder joint, and the clavicular fibers of the pectoralis major); and (b) the triceps brachii (elbow extensor). While standing with the feet shoulder-width apart, pick up a 2- to 3-lb dumbbell and position it at the shoulders while keeping the wrist straight. Breathe in as the dumbbell is pushed over the head until the arm is fully flexed at the shoulder and extended at the elbow. A small arch in the low back will help in positioning the weight straight overhead. Then, breathe out as the dumbbell is lowered to the shoulder. Repeat the exercise 10 times to complete 1 set. Rest for 1 min and start the second set of 10 repetitions.

The **Dumbbell Squat** is the third resistance training exercise. The squat exercise strengthens the thighs and buttocks. At the thigh, the quadriceps consist of four muscles: (a) vastus lateralis, (b) vastus medialis, (c) vastus intermedius, and (d) rectus femoris. At the buttocks, the *gluteal muscles* are a group of three *muscles*: (a) *gluteus* maximus, (b) *gluteus* medius, and (c) *gluteus* minimus. To begin the exercise, take two dumbbells (one in each hand). Assume an upright standing position and start exhaling during the squat until the thighs are close to a horizontal position (or as low as is comfortable). Keep the head, shoulders, and chest upright entering into the squat position, which is controlled by the eccentric contraction of the gluteal, hamstring, and quadriceps muscles. Start inhaling during the standing part of the exercise and exhaling during the flexing of the hips and knees. The concentric contraction of quadriceps muscles and the gluteal muscles extend the knees and hips, respectively.

The fourth resistance training exercise is the **Dumbbell Calf Raise**. This exercise strengthens the gastrocnemius and soleus muscles that are responsible for plantar flexion, which is movement of the foot and toes away from the body. When walking, they contract to provide a force against the ground to keep the ankle in a normal position when the body's weight is over the foot. Although it is common for both hands to hold a dumbbell while both feet undergo plantar flexion, it is safer for the elderly frail adult to work one calf at a time while maintaining balance by holding the back of a chair during the exercise.

To begin, hold the dumbbell on the side of the calf being exercised (e.g., with the dumbbell in the right hand, do a calf raise with the right leg). Stand with the toes on a 2- to 3-inch board to position the ankle in a slight dorsiflexed position, which will place the calf muscles in a slightly stretched position to intensify the concentric (shortening) contraction. Using a 3- to 5-lb dumbbell, press the front part of the foot against the board and body will rise as the ankle undergoes plantar flexion. Do 8 to 12 repetitions (1 set), rest for 1 min, and then do a second set before moving to the other side of the body to repeat the sequence. Don't forget to inhale on the way up on tiptoe and exhale as the heel is lowered to the floor.

The fifth and final resistance training exercise is the **Dumbbell Row**, which helps to strengthen primarily the posterior and middle deltoids and the long head of the triceps brachii. Other muscles (e.g., infraspinatus, teres major, and teres minor) that cross the shoulder joint are not as strong at extending or hyperextending the shoulder, given that they primarily protect the integrity of the shoulder joint as rotator cuff muscles.

This exercise is typically performed with the hips flexed at 90°. But that is not the case with the elderly frail adult. At ~45° angle, the hip position is sufficient to allow the exercise to be performed safely while holding the top of a chair with one hand in front of the body. The other hand is used to hold the dumbbell while bending forward. The dumbbell is pulled up (producing shoulder extension and hyperextension as well as elbow flexion) to touch the side of the waist. Then, it is slowly lowered to the original position. Inhale as the weight is pulled up and exhale as the weight is lowered. Using a 2- to 3-lb dumbbell, do 8 to 10 repetitions (set 1) followed by a 1-min rest prior to set 2.

## Final Thoughts

Do the five resistance training exercises twice weekly. Doing the exercises one time a week will not produce the desired results. Resistance training will result in some soreness, so the elderly frail adults should be aware that soreness is normal. Most of the soreness and aches will subside within a day or two. It is important to rest a full day between the exercise sessions (e.g., rest on Wednesday if it is a Tuesday and Thursday schedule). The complete program is threefold: (a) resistance training, (b) flexibility training, and (c) aerobic training.

While aging is a natural process, the changes in the body and mind that produce various issues if not problems demand the attention of Exercise Physiologists who believe in Jesus Christ as the Son of God. After all, positive beliefs and strength are gained from our thoughts, experiences, and prayer, all of which can contribute to the patient or client's well-being (Akbari 2018). Elizabeth Scott (2020) said it best,

> While people use many different religions and paths to find God or to express their spirituality, research has shown that those who are more religious or spiritual and use their spirituality to cope with life experience many benefits to their health and well-being.

It may even promote healing. This is especially the case with the increase in the elderly population. The importance of the exercise physiology profession in counseling and prescribing exercise medicine is to highlight ASEP's role in the academic accreditation of exercise physiology. The ASEP exercise physiologists understand the musculoskeletal system and the specifics of resistance training to bring about improvements in balance and a decrease in falls and hospitalization.

## References

Akbari M, Hossaini SM. (2018). Mental Health, and Burnout: The Mediating Role of Emotional Regulation. *Iranian Journal of Psychiatry*. 13(1);22–31.

Chodzko-Zajko, WJ, Proctor, DN, Fiatarone-Singh, MA, et al. (2009). American College of Sports Medicine Position Stand. Exercise and Physical Activity for Older Adults. *Medicine & Science in Sports & Exercise*. 41(7);1510–1530.

Cooper, R, Kuh, D, Hardy, R. (2010). Objectively Measured of Physical Capability Levels and Mortality: Systematic Review and Meta-Analysis. *British Medical Journal.* 9(341);4467.

Duren, DL, Sherwood, RJ, Czerwinski, SA, et al. (2008). Body Composition Methods: Comparisons and Interpretation. *Journal of Diabetes Science and Technology.* 2(6);1139–1146.

Frontera, WR, Meredith, CN, O'Reilly, KP, Knuttgen, HG, Evans, WJ. (1988). Strength Conditioning in Older Men: Skeletal Muscle Hypertrophy and Improved Function. *Journal of Applied Physiology.* 64;1038–1044.

Goodpaster, BH, Park, SW, Harris, TB, et al. (2006). The Loss of Skeletal Muscle Strength, Mass, and Quality in Older Adults: The Health, Aging and body Composition Study. *Journal of Gerontology. A Biological Science and Medical Science.* 61;1059–1064.

Hughes, VA, Frontera, WR, Wood, M, et al. (2001). Longitudinal Muscle Strength Changes in Older Adults: Influence of Muscle Mass, Physical Activity, and Health. *Journal of Gerontology. A Biological Science and Medical Science.* 56;209–217.

Kirkendall, DT, Garrett, WE, Jr. (1998). The Effects of Aging and Training on Skeletal Muscle. *American Journal of Sports Medicine.* 26;598–602.

Paneni, F, Canestro, CD, Libby, P, et al. (2017). The Aging Cardiovascular System: Understanding it at the Cellular and Clinical Levels. *Journal of the American College of Cardiology.* 69(15);1952–1967.

Scott, E. (2020). *How Spirituality Can Benefit Mental and Physical Health* [Online]. www.verywellmind.com/how-spirituality-can-benefit-mental-and-physical-health-3144807

# 10

# FLEXIBILITY TRAINING AND FRAIL ADULTS

The range of motion in the joints throughout the body decreases with aging, poor physical health, and a sedentary lifestyle. The primary reason for the decrease in flexibility in the pre-frail and frail older adults is due to the changes in the skeletal muscles that result in low muscle function and deterioration in movement. Moreover, the age-related loss in muscle size (e.g., the vastus lateralis by up to 40% between 20 and 80 years of age) is a risk factor for disability, hospitalization, and death in older adults (Fielding et al. 2011; Lexell 1995).

It is important that ASEP Board-Certified Exercise Physiologists recommend and assist in the identification of specific muscle building and flexibility exercises (Boone 2016). Doing so, especially in conjunction with resistance exercises and aerobic training will set the stage for a higher level of physical functioning with a decrease in physical disabilities that are linked to the decrease in range of motion. Also, the decrease in age-related muscle loss will result in a major savings in healthcare costs (Janssen et al. 2004).

Aside from the common expectation of athletes and non-athletes to warm-up by stretching their muscles, having adequate flexibility is a major healthcare concern. Unfortunately, athletes and adults of all ages who do engage in stretching exercises do not understand that many of the exercises are of no value or the exercises are potentially dangerous for the involved joints (Boone 2017). Yet, with the "right flexibility exercises," posture, balance, and range of motion can be improved with a decrease in the likelihood of falling and suffering an injury.

## Frail Adults Have Similar Flexibility Needs

What is not well understood is that elderly frail adults need a normal range of muscle and joint flexibility just as middle-aged adults do. In fact, Speer (2005) indicates that flexibility exercises are a major part of a rehabilitation program to help adult patients with a history of chronic diseases, disabilities (i.e., limitation in the ability to perform basic functional activities), and injuries that often restrict range of motion while increasing healthcare costs (Chan et al. 2002). Consequently, for the majority of the frail adults and the elderly frail adults in community dwellings and assisted living homes, the goal is to increase range of motion in hip flexion and extension muscles and in the shoulder extension and hyperextension muscles to allow for an unrestricted range of motion in daily activities.

DOI: 10.4324/9781003119920-13

---

**BOX 10.1  FLEXIBILITY IMPROVEMENT AND AGING.**

"While joint flexibility may decrease with age, with the potential to affect normal daily function, older adults do maintain the ability to improve flexibility through stretching exercises."

—Paterson, DH, Warburton, DER. (2010). Physical Activity and Functional Limitations in Older Adults: A Systematic Review Related to Canada's Physical Activity guidelines. *International Journal of Behavioral Nutrition and Physical Activity.* 7;38.

---

The design of the flexibility program is the same regardless of the person's age, gender, and/or range of motion. Both middle-aged and elderly adults should concentrate on the same exercises. To do differently is not only unnecessary but also a waste of time. Also, the use of flexibility exercises that are potentially dangerous to the ligaments, tendons, and cartilage at certain joints must be avoided.

Hence, the more the flexibility exercises, the better is not the correct approach to increasing range of motion. It is unfortunately the result of a poor understanding of the anatomy of the body. Instructors who encourage their clients to do a dozen or more stretching exercises are prone to including not only useless but also dangerous exercises. Hence, as hard as it might be to believe, only "three" slow-stretching exercises are necessary to increase the range of motion of the major muscle groups throughout the body.

It is also a waste of time to do a stretching exercise to increase the range of motion of a joint that already has a maximal range of movement. Such exercises are meaningless. Instead, why not engage in stretching exercises at joints where there is a limitation in the range of motion? For example, why not train to increase the range of hyperextension of the shoulder muscles and the hip muscles of most elderly frail adults? The insertion of the pectoralis major on the lateral lip of the bicipital groove not only limits extension and hyperextension but also inwardly rotates the arm while creating a constant state of shoulder flexion that encourages adaptive shortening. This is common among aging adults who also live with adaptive shortening of the hip flexors that result in a forward inclination of the upper body.

## The "Three" Good Flexibility Exercises

### Number 1: Sit–Straddle–Reach Stretch

From the sitting position on the floor, the "Sit–Straddle–Reach" exercise begins with the legs abducted (i.e., spread as wide as possible). It is the best exercise to increase range of motion of the low back, hamstring, and adductor muscles. Relax while stretching and do not bounce or use force in moving the hands toward the feet. Also, the feet should be in the dorsiflexed position (i.e., with the toes and feet pointed back toward the upper body) when leaning forward to help with stretching the calf muscles of the posterior leg (i.e., in particular, the gastrocnemius and soleus).

Remember to inhale at the start of the exercise and exhale gradually during the slow stretch forward of the chest over the thigh followed by a hold position. During the first week of stretching, hold the stretch for a short period of time (e.g., 3 to 5 sec). Repeat each stretch

three times during each of the three sessions (such as MWF), first over the right thigh followed by stretching over the left thigh. By the second week, the duration of the stretch can be
increased 10 sec repeated two times in each session. During the third week, the stretch should
be increased to ~20 sec each (repeated two times each). By the fourth week, hold the stretch
~30 sec. Each stretch should be repeated three times. It is a good flexibility exercise because it
is safe and because the tension placed on the erector spinae (low back muscles) and hamstring
muscles (located on the posterior thigh) is under the elderly adult's control.

This exercise counteracts the adaptive shortening that occurs with years of sitting and physical inactivity that decreases the range of motion of the erector spinae, hamstrings, adductors,
and plantar flexors. The increase in anterior convexity of the spine while sitting allows for
shortening of the low back muscles, which often results in low back pain. The flexed position
of the knees along with the legs held close together promotes shortening of the hamstrings
and the adductors of the thigh. The Sit–Straddle–Reach is an excellent exercise to stretch
the erector spinae muscles of the back. To gain full benefit of the stretch, keep the lumbar
and thoracic areas as straight as possible when leaning forward (i.e., while flexing at the hips).
Although there will be a natural roundness of the mid-thoracic region, it is best to keep the
back as straight as possible.

The semitendinosus muscle is the first of the three hamstring muscles. It arises from the
superior lateral surface of the ischial tuberosity to insert into the proximal medial condyle of
the tibia. The signature design of the muscle is its palpable tendon of insertion. The semitendinosus extends, hyperextends, and adducts the thigh at the hip joint. At the knee joint,
it flexes and medially rotates the tibia. The semimembranosus arises from the upper outer
quadrant of poster surface of ischial tuberosity. It inserts with the semitendinosus muscle on
the proximal medial condyle of the tibia. The third hamstring muscle is the long head of the
biceps femoris, which arises along with the semitendinosus from the ischial tuberosity to
insert into the head of the fibula with a small slip to the lateral condyle of the tibia. All three
muscles are innervated by the medial division of the sciatic nerve.

The long head of the biceps femoris extends, hyperextends, and adducts the thigh at the
hip joint while flexing the knee joint. The short head of the biceps femoris arises from the
lateral lip of the linea aspera and part of the lateral supracondylar ridge to insert as a common
tendon with the long head. The short head is innervated by the lateral division of the sciatic
nerve (otherwise referred to as the common peroneal nerve). The short head of biceps femoris flexes the knee joint. It also laterally rotates the tibia with help from the long head. It is the
only hamstring muscle innervated by two nerves.

The powerhouse muscle that helps the hamstrings at the hip joint is the vertical fibers of
the adductor magnus. It arises from the lateral aspect of the ischial tuberosity and the inferior
surface of the ischium to insert into the full length of the medial lip of the linea aspera, medial
supracondylar ridge, and the adductor tubercle. It is a one-joint muscle that produces hip
extension and hyperextension.

The pectineus muscle (usually identified as the first of the five adductor muscles of the
medial thigh) is a flat, quadrangular muscle. It arises from the anterior, superior border of
the pubic bone to insert into the pectineal line, which is just inferior to the lesser trochanter
of the femur. The pectineus muscle flexes the hip joint, and it can also adduct and externally
rotate the thigh. The pectineus is innervated by the femoral nerve, which arises from the
anterior horns of spinal segments L2–L4 of the lumbar plexus.

The adductor longus is the second muscle of the medial thigh (i.e., from lateral to medial). It arises from the anterior upper one-half of the symphysis pubis to insert into the middle one-third of the medial lip of the linea aspera (i.e., an osteological bony projection on the dorsal medial surface of the femur from the lesser tuberosity to the medial supracondylar ridge). The adductor longus flexes the hip joint. It also adducts and laterally rotates the thigh. It is innervated by the obturator nerve that arises from the anterior horns of spinal segments L2–L4 of the lumbar plexus.

## BOX 10.2   THE ADDUCTOR MUSCLES OF THE HIP AND THIGH (BOONE 2017, ANATOMY).

Psoas Major     Iliacus     Adductor Longus     Adductor Magnus

Pectineus     Adductor Brevis     Gracilis

The adductor brevis muscle arises from the inferior border of the pubic bone to insert into the upper one-half of the medial lip of the linea aspera. It flexes the hip joint, adducts, and laterally rotates the thigh. Anatomically, from the anterior perspective, the adductor brevis is located posterior to the adductor longus. It is innervated by the obturator nerve.

The anterior fibers of the adductor magnus arise from the inferior lateral border of the pubic bone. Collectively, the fibers insert on the upper medial lip of the linea aspera, which approximates the pectineal line. Functionally, it is more like the adductor brevis muscle than the adductor magnus (vertical fibers) muscle. The anterior fibers of the adductor magnus are innervated by the obturator nerve, which arises from the ventral divisions of the second, third, and fourth lumbar nerves in the lumbar plexus.

The least stretched muscles of the lower back, the hamstrings, the adductors, and the plantar flexors are the muscles that cross the ankle joint to plantar flex the foot. There are six plantar flexors in the posterior compartment of the leg and two in the lateral compartment of the leg. The six muscles are innervated by the tibial nerve, which is the distal part of the medial division of the sciatic nerve. The two muscles that originate from within the lateral compartment of the leg are innervated by the superficial branch of the common peroneal nerve.

The muscles in the posterior compartment are arranged in two layers, superficial and deep. The superficial layer is made up of three muscles, from superficial to deep, they are gastrocnemius, plantaris, and soleus. The first two are two-joint muscles. The soleus is a one-joint muscle. The plantaris is the weakest of the plantar flexors, while the soleus is the strongest of the three in the superficial layer and the strongest of the eight altogether. The gastrocnemius flexes the knee, and plantar flexes the foot. If the knee is flexed, it is not as strong as the ankle joint. The plantaris is 90% tendon and, therefore, without sufficient muscle size to produce a strong force. It is a very weak flexor of the knee and ankle joints.

The gastrocnemius arises from the medial and lateral condyles of the femur to insert into the dorsal surface of the calcaneus (heel bone). The plantaris arises from the lateral epicondyle of the femur to insert into the more medial side of the dorsal surface of the calcaneus. The soleus arises from the proximal dorsal two-thirds of the fibula and tibia to insert into the dorsal surface of the calcaneus.

The plantar flexor muscles of the deep layer are commonly identified from medial to lateral. They are the flexor hallucis longus, the tibialis posterior, and the flexor digitorum longus muscles. All three muscles exit the posterior, deep layer of the leg by way of the medial malleolus. The flexor hallucis longus arises from the dorsal distal two-thirds of the fibula to insert via the plantar surface of the distal phalanx of digit #1. Its plantar flexes and/or inverts the ankle joint while flexing the big toe.

The tibialis posterior muscle arises from the proximal dorsal two-thirds of the fibula, tibia, and the intervening interosseous membrane. The muscle inserts by way of the plantar surface of the navicular tuberosity. Its primary responsibility, aside from plantar flexion and inversion, is to support the arch of the foot. The flexor digitorum longus arises from the dorsal distal two-thirds of the tibia and inserts via the plantar surfaces of the distal phalanges, digits 2 to 5. The flexor digitorum longus plantar flexes and inverts the ankle joint. It is also the primary flexors of digits 2 through 5.

When the foot is dorsiflexed, as during the standing wall stretch, it tends to place a stretch on these six muscles in the dorsal compartment of the leg, and the two muscles that arise from within the lateral compartment of the leg. The peroneus longus (also known as fibularis longus) arises from the upper one-half of the lateral surface of the fibula, and the peroneus brevis (also known as the fibularis brevis) arises from the lower one-half of the lateral surface of the fibula (Nelson & Kokkonen 2007).

The peroneus longus ends with a long tendon that runs dorsal to the lateral malleolus to insert into the inferior surfaces of bones on the medial side of the foot, but specifically on the lateral side of the base of the first metatarsal and the lateral-distal end of the medial cuneiform #2. The peroneus brevis also passes dorsal to the lateral malleolus to insert into the dorsal surface of the base of the fifth metatarsal (i.e., the metatarsal that gives rise to the little toe).

Both the peroneus longus and peroneus brevis work with the six primary plantar flexors of the foot and ankle joint (i.e., the gastrocnemius and soleus). Of the two posterior leg muscles, the soleus is the most powerful plantar flexor, given that it is a one-joint muscle at the ankle.

## Number 2: Shoulder and Chest Stretch

The "Shoulder and Chest" stretch is the second of the three good flexibility exercises. It is important for several reasons. The primary concern is the influence of a sedentary lifestyle on the shoulder and chest muscles that undergo atrophy, loss of strength, and flexibility. Also, the lack of regular exercise and the predisposition of the upper limbs in the forward position (as when sitting at a desk typing for hours) minimizes the stretch placed on the muscles of the anterior shoulder and chest. The result is a decrease in the normal range of motion, which predisposes to a forward inclination of the shoulders and the tendency to abduct the scapula and round out the upper back.

The shoulder and chest muscles that are stretched during this exercise are the pectoralis major, pectoralis minor, anterior deltoid, coracobrachialis, and the short and long heads of the biceps brachii. Aside from the pectoralis minor that inserts onto the coracoid process and the sternocostal fibers of the pectoralis major, the remaining muscles are the primary should flexors.

By placing the upper limbs behind the body while sitting and, then, moving the hips forward (as the hips and knees are flexed), the shoulders will undergo hyperextension. The body position will result in a progressive increase in the stretching of the shoulder flexors. This is important because the shortening of the shoulder flexors limits the range of motion of the upper limbs along with the tendency of the shoulders to move forward while the arms inwardly rotate. The newly acquired rounding of the shoulders alters the respiratory activity with a resultant decrease in efficiency of the upper extremities and breathing.

The clavicular fibers of the pectoralis major arise from the proximal anterior one-half of the clavicle. The fibers converge to insert into the proximal lateral lip of the bicipital groove with the fibers from the sternal part of the muscle. Both functional parts of the pectoralis major adduct and inwardly rotate the arm. The clavicular fibers flex and abduct the arm while the sternocostal fibers extend and adduct the arm. The clavicular fibers are innervated by the lateral pectoral nerve (C5, C6), while the sternocostal fibers are innervated by the medial pectoral nerve (C7, C8, T1).

Arising from the anterior distal one-third of the clavicle is the anterior deltoid. The middle deltoid arises from the acromion process of the scapula. The posterior deltoid arises from the spine of the scapula. The three muscles insert via the deltoid tuberosity of the humerus. The anterior deltoid is a shoulder flexor and inward rotator of the arm. The posterior deltoid is a shoulder extensor and outward rotator of the arm. The middle deltoid works with both the anterior and posterior deltoid muscles. It is the strongest of the three in abducting the arm. The deltoid muscle is innervated by the axillary nerve.

Deep to the pectoralis major and anterior deltoid are two muscles. They are the coraco-brachialis and the short head of the biceps brachii. Both muscles are innervated by the mus-culocutaneous nerve. They work together to flex, inwardly rotate, and adduct the humerus. When the origin and insertion move close to each other, as in sitting with the arms in front of the chest, the muscles tend to undergo adaptive shortening. To counteract the loss in range of motion in the shoulder joints, the "shoulder and chest stretch" helps to maintain or increase the flexibility of the shoulder flexors.

---

**BOX 10.3  CORACOBRACHIALIS (A) AND SHORT HEAD OF THE BICEPS BRACHII (B) IN DARK ON THE MEDIAL SIDE AND THE PECTORALIS MINOR ARISING FROM OUTER SURFACE OF RIBS 3 TO 5.**

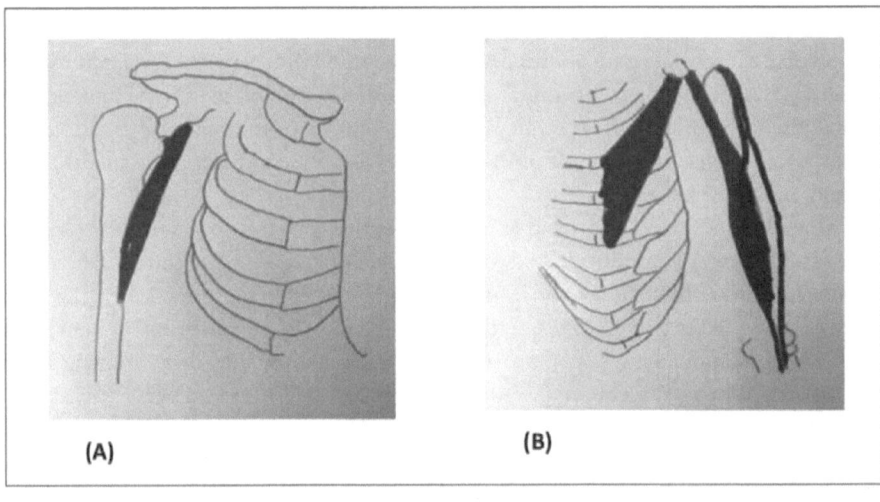

(A)                                                    (B)

---

### Number 3: Standing Hip Flexor Stretch

The third exercise of the three good flexibility exercises is the "Standing Hip Flexor Stretch." One foot is placed forward with the knee over the foot. The other foot is placed behind the body. Note that the upper body is vertical from the head through the hips, which is an important body position. If the chest is positioned forward to a position essentially over the flexed knee, the hip flexors on the straight leg side will not be stretched. With the head and shoulders in the vertical position, the back foot is moved a few inches backward to place a greater stretch on the hip flexors. Then, the exercise is repeated on the other side of the body.

The psoas major, iliacus, tensor fascia latae, gluteus medius (anterior fibers), gluteus mini-mus (anterior fibers), sartorius, and rectus femoris are the primary muscles stretched during the hip flexor stretch exercise. The secondary muscles stretched are the pectineus, adductor longus, gracilis, adductor brevis, and adductor magnus (anterior fibers). Aside from these muscles acting primarily as hip adductors, they also flex the hip. The hip flexor stretch is an excellent exercise to increase the range of motion of all 12 muscles.

The psoas major muscle arises from the five transverse processes and sides of the lumbar vertebrae to insert along with the iliacus muscle via the lesser trochanter. The iliacus arises from the anterior fossa of the ilium. Both muscles are innervated by the femoral nerve of the lumbar plexus. They are also known as the iliopsoas muscle since they function as one muscle to flex the hip, adduct the thigh, and outwardly rotate the femur.

The tensor fascia latae arises from the anterior superior iliac spine (ASIS). It inserts via the upper one-fourth of the iliotibial tract (also known as the fascia lata). The tensor fascia latae assists in flexing and internally rotating the thigh. It also abducts the lower limb, extends the knee, and laterally rotates the leg. It is innervated by the superior gluteal nerve, which also innervates the gluteus medius and the gluteus minimus muscles.

The gluteus medius and gluteus minimus originate from the upper posterior surface of the ilium. Aside from their primary action of abduction of the hip joint (along with the tensor fascia latae), the anterior part of each muscle is responsible for flexing the hip joint and inwardly rotating the thigh. The posterior part of both muscles extends the thigh and outwardly rotates the lower limb.

The sartorius also arises from the ASIS. It inserts on the tibia in essentially the same place as the gracilis muscle, although slightly more anterior on the tibia. Like the tensor fascia latae, the sartorius flexes the hip, laterally rotates the thigh, and flexes the knee joint. It can also rotate the tibia medially (along with the gracilis) when the knee is flexed. The sartorius is innervated by the femoral nerve.

Just below the ASIS is the anterior inferior iliac spine. It is the origin of the rectus femoris. The muscle gets its name from the fascicle orientation (*rectus* = straight). It is the most superficial muscle in the anterior compartment of the thigh. The rectus femoris inserts on the tibia tuberosity (i.e., the anterior proximal aspect of the tibia) via the patellar ligament and quadriceps tendon. The rectus femoris is primarily a knee extensor, but it will also flex the hip and abduct the lower limb if the thigh is laterally rotated first. It is innervated by the femoral nerve, which is one of the major nerves supplying the lower limb.

## Final Thoughts

The majority of adults who work in coaching, fitness, athletics, sports medicine, and the medical community are not aware that there are good, useless, and dangerous flexibility exercises. While the "good" exercises result in a tremendous benefit to the musculoskeletal system, the "useless" exercises are a waste of time because the muscles seldom need stretching. The "dangerous" exercises can and often do result in an injury to the muscles and tendons. These exercises are explained in more detail in *Anatomy: A Pressing Concern in Exercise Physiology*.

If athletes were to use just the "three good exercises" described in this chapter, they would have more time to optimize their full range of motion throughout the body. In fact, these exercises are sufficient to develop the flexibility needed by gymnasts to perform their gymnastic routines. Given that this is the case with gymnasts who need a greater range of motion than the majority of athletes in dozens of different sports, it should be obvious that (a) the **sit–straddle–reach stretch,** (b) the **shoulder and chest stretch**, and (c) the **standing hip flexor stretch** constitute a complete flexibility program for the elderly frail adults to develop and/or maintain their range of motion throughout the body.

**BOX 10.4   THIS BOOK EXPLAINS THE ANATOMICAL SPECIFICS OF THE GOOD, USELESS, AND DANGEROUS FLEXIBILITY EXERCISES.**

eISBN: 978-1-68108-469-5
ISBN:  978-1-68108-470-1

ANATOMY:
A PRESSING CONCERN IN EXERCISE PHYSIOLOGY
COMMITMENT TO PROFESSIONALISM

Tommy Boone

Bentham Books

While the "Anatomy" book was written from the ASEP perspective to clarify the importance of understanding both anatomy and physiology of the body, it was also written specifically for the ASEP Board-Certified Exercise Physiologists. They are recognized as certified healthcare professionals with a strong academic background in the anatomy of fitness, physical activity, and exercise medicine. They are in a great position to work with patients referred to them by a healthcare provider to assess the patient's physical activity with the expectation of providing an exercise medicine prescription (Boone 2015, 2016).

## References

Boone, T. (2015). *Promoting Professionalism in Exercise Physiology: Vision, Challenges, and Opportunities.* Lewiston, NY: The Edwin Mellen Press.

Boone, T. (2016). *ASEP's Exercise Medicine Text for Exercise Physiologists*. Sharjah, UAE: Bentham Science Publishers.

Boone, T. (2017). *Anatomy: A Pressing Concern in Exercise Physiology*. Sharjah, UAE: Bentham Science Publishers.

Chan, L, Beaver, S, Maclehose, RF, et al. (2002). Disability and Health Care Costs in the Medicare Population. *Archives of Physical Medicine and Rehabilitation*. 83(9);1196–1201.

Fielding, RA, Vellas, B, Evans, WJ, et al. (2011). Sarcopenia: An Undiagnosed Condition in Older Adults. Current Consensus Definition: Prevalence, Etiology, and Consequences. International Working Group on Sarcopenia. *Journal of the American Medical Directors Association*. 12;249–256.

Janssen, I, Shepard, DS, Katzmarzyk, PT, Roubenoff, R. (2004). The Healthcare Costs of Sarcopenia in the United States. *Journal of the American Geriatric Society*. 52;80–85.

Lexell, J. (1995). Human Aging, Muscle Mass, and Fiber Type Composition. *Journals of Gerontology. Series A, Biological Sciences and Medical Sciences*. 50;11–16.

Nelson, AG, Kokkonen, J. (2007). *Stretching Anatomy*. Champaign, IL: Human Kinetics Publishers.

Paterson, DH, Warburton, DER. (2010). Physical Activity and Functional Limitations in Older Adults: A Systematic Review Related to Canada's Physical Activity Guidelines. *International Journal of Behavioral Nutrition and Physical Activity*. 7;38.

Speer, KP. (2005). *Injury Prevention and Rehabilitation for Active Older Adults*. Champaign, IL: Human Kinetics Publishers.

# 11

# AEROBIC TRAINING AND FRAIL ADULTS

The clock is ticking. Men and women are getting older, and many have avoided being physically active. In fact, according to Steve Blair (2009), "Physical inactivity is the biggest public health problem of the 21st century." The physiological changes in the body are consistent with a diminished aerobic capacity that is associated with fatigue and breathlessness. The number of oxygen-carrying red blood cells decreases with aging. There is a decrease in muscle size, strength, and bone density, and yet the body is larger than it should be due to the increase in fat that contributes to the increase in LDL cholesterol and the decrease in HDL cholesterol. Blood sugar levels increase, making the likelihood of type 2 diabetes a reality among aging adults (Boone 2014, 2016). There are also changes in the nervous system with aging.

While regular exercise cannot stop the aging process, it can slow it down. After all, a major contributor to an earlier onset of the effects of aging is a sedentary lifestyle. Also, it is important to note that older adults respond nearly as well to an exercise medicine prescription as they would have at the age of 30. The human body can benefit from exercise at any age. Aging is inevitable, but regular exercise can slow the aging process. It is never too late to do a daily 10-min warm-up followed by a 20- or 30-min walk and cool down.

The interaction between exercise and aging is dramatic, especially since it can be used to treat and prevent many chronic conditions. An exercise medicine program can correct the physiological alterations that occur during periods of physical inactivity. Regular exercise can contribute to improvements in health and well-being by helping to control the development of chronic diseases that increases life expectancy, and by helping to prevent age-related disorders. After all, essentially every part of the body is influenced in a positive way by exercise.

Hence, it is important that elderly frail adults become physically active to decrease their risk of harmful health effects from heart disease, pulmonary disease, type 2 diabetes, obesity, and colon cancer (Ciolac 2013). Also, according to Schuch et al. (2018), living a physically inactive lifestyle is linked to mental depression that affects 17 million Americans along with other negative mental outcomes.

DOI: 10.4324/9781003119920-14

## BOX 11.1  THE DALLAS BED REST AND TRAINING STUDY.

In 1966, five healthy men volunteered for a research study at the University of Texas Southwestern Medical School. Prior to the subjects spending 3 weeks resting in bed, they were tested for aerobic capacity. When they got out of the bed at the end of the 3-week period, the researchers tested them again. They found that the subjects had a faster resting heart rate, higher systolic blood pressure, a decrease in the heart's maximum pumping capacity, an increase in body fat, and a decrease in muscle strength.

—Saltin, B, Blomqvist, G, Mitchell, JH, et al. (1968). Response to Exercise After Bed Rest and After Training. *Circulation*. 38(5);VIII–VII78.

Participation in an exercise medicine program increases cardiorespiratory fitness. The higher the cardiorespiratory capacity of the aging adult, the lower the risk for mortality (Blair et al. 1989), whereas a lower level of cardiorespiratory fitness increases mortality risk. In fact, Lee et al. (2012) reported, "If inactivity decreased by 25%, more than 1.3 million deaths worldwide could be averted every year."

## BOX 11.2  CLINICAL CONSEQUENCES OF A LIFETIME OF PHYSICAL INACTIVITY.

"Clinical consequences that arise from the accelerated decrease in $VO_2$ max due to a lifetime of physical inactivity are: (a) increased mortality so death occurs at an earlier age; (b) younger age for the onset of physical frailty; (c) fewer years of high quality of life; (d) lowered cardiorespiratory reserve so that stresses, such as major surgery, are insufficient to maintain homeostasis within bounds of life; and (5) increased risk of chronic diseases."

—Booth, FW, Laye, MJ, Roberts, MD. (2011). Lifetime Sedentary Living Accelerates Some Aspects of Secondary Aging. *Journal of Applied Physiology*. 111(5);1497–1504.

Participation in lifelong aerobic exercise results in a delay in physical dependency and more years with a good quality of life. With a higher than average level of functional capacity, adults who are 60 to 80 years of age will have an increased tolerance for physiologically stressful situations (such as a major surgery). Hence, older adults with a high cardiorespiratory fitness level will be mentally and physically better prepared to avoid morbidity and mortality (Struthers et al. 2008). In fact, regular exercise is even more effective than medication in the rehabilitation of patients after a stroke (Naci & Ioannidis 2015).

With these life-saving health benefits, why wouldn't middle-aged adults and aging elderly adults schedule time to go for a 20- to 30-min walk at a frequency of 3 to 5 days a week? Or, they could benefit as well by exercising on a cycle-ergometer or by engaging in water-based exercises to improve cardiovascular function and their quality of life during aging. The bottom line is that aerobic exercise training will either maintain or improve the elderly adult's cardiac function by keeping the myocardium supple and the arteries flexible with a lower resting heart rate and blood pressure, as well as an increase in the heart's ability to deliver oxygen-rich blood to the body's tissues.

---

### BOX 11.3   DEFINITION OF AEROBIC EXERCISE.

A 10-min brisk walk will make the heart and cardiovascular system stronger, which lead to improved mental focus and clarity, and reduced stress. Repeating the walk 2 or 3 times·d$^{-1}$ will make the muscles stronger and more flexible.

---

The key to a healthier life for the elderly frail adults is regular exercise. Aging adults can avoid frailty and protect the body's metabolism from the effects of aging, improve sleep, boosts mood, and avoid age-related memory loss. Simply by taking the advice of an ASEP Board-Certified Exercise Physiologist, aging adults can protect the body and mind by starting slowly and building up gradually to enjoy a 30-min brisk walk nearly every day of the week. As Thompson and colleagues (2020) pointed out,

> Exercise is a medicine that can prevent and treat chronic disease; those who take it live longer and with a higher quality of life." Hence, it is imperative that adults, frail or otherwise, keep moving. As Hippocrates said 2,400 years ago, "That which is used develops; that which is not wastes away.

## Exercise Precautions

For an exercise medicine prescription to be safe and properly carried out, healthcare providers should refer their patients to an ASEP Board-Certified Exercise Physiologist as part of every patient's treatment plan. Hence, following the elderly frail adults' medical check-ups and screening, the ASEP exercise physiologist will initiate a cardiovascular assessment prior to starting an exercise program. The screening will include a personal history of the adult's cardiovascular, pulmonary, or metabolic disease, identification of risk factors, a submaximal exercise ECG, blood pressure, and $VO_2$ to identify the potential for cardiovascular benefits and problems as well as the beginning point for starting the low-to-moderate-intensity exercise medicine program. Periodic physiologic testing will be part of the program protocol, particularly with respect to monitoring the effectiveness of the exercise prescription. Of course, it is important that the prescription process is also educational with appropriate time spent to clarify the targeted effects of the training program on mind–body improvements.

Aging adults frequently encounter unanticipated questions and challenges in training. These include unexplained reasons for a specific exercise program or a combination of programs and/or the failure to understand the training effect on different physiologic factors. Thus, the exercise prescription as exercise medicine will have an educational component that explains the anticipated changes in the aging adult's physiologic profile. For example, if the elderly frail adult's economy of movement is significantly decreased, then emphasis on training techniques that are expected to improve specific physiologic variables while explaining the role of the variables that reduce or increase efficiency is appropriate.

---

**BOX 11.4  DEFINITION OF FRAILTY.**

Frailty is a common clinical syndrome in older adults that carries an increased risk for poor health outcomes including falls, incident disability, hospitalization, and mortality.

---

In other words, aside from understanding that exercise progression is a function of frequency, intensity, and duration, ASEP Board-Certified Exercise Physiologists also understand the importance of educating and troubleshooting the adult's health problems that are linked to aging and frailty. The continued demand for an economically sound and physiologically evidence-based proven medicine in the form of regular exercise requires that exercise physiologists and medical practitioners work together to optimize the frail adults' health and exercise performance. But, having said that, it is important that the profession of exercise physiology continues to promote and prescribe regular exercise as a personalized medicine. This means optimizing exercise dosing strategies per adult to maximize health benefits while also minimizing psychological and lifestyle barriers to participation. This is done by increasing the educational relevance of anatomical and physiological changes that result from exercise medicine as therapy.

Such work by exercise physiologists will continue to have a strong influence not only on the improvement of healthcare outcomes but also on the exercise physiology profession. Such targeted thinking and exercise medicine interventions combined with nutritional and other forms of counseling and therapy (such as progressive relaxation techniques) will help to improve the patient's training results. In addition, exercise physiologists have not investigated the effects of interventions that use spirituality and home-based exercise as well as entrepreneur-based exercise strategies to optimize the beneficial effects of personalized exercise regimens and career opportunities. Yet it is common knowledge that less than one-third of all doctors advised their patients to engage in regular exercise. Almost assuredly, far fewer have taken an active role in prescribing exercise to their patients as well as speaking to the role of spirituality in exercise medicine programs.

The ASEP organization is poised to promote and build upon this thinking to enhance dialogue and exchange of ideas to increase the involvement of exercise physiologists in the overall health assessment and well-being of target populations. Hence, there isn't any question that regular exercise should be considered a viable alternative to or in combination with specific medications. While it is tempting to believe that popping an exercise pill will cure all the ills of aging adults, that isn't the case at all. Instead, rather basic healthy lifestyle changes (such as being physically active and eating well) have proven effective in improving mental and physical well-being.

---

**BOX 11.5  WHEN IS AN "EXERCISE PILL" A GOOD THING?**

What about people who are injured? Or, what about people who can't exercise or who have a genetic disorder that prevents them from building lean muscle mass and having the musculoskeletal system to safely engage in regular exercise? With an exercise pill, they could reap the benefits of the exercise their bodies won't let them do, that is, if it is true that an injury lasts a lifetime or if there is a genetic disorder that prevents a person from participating in an individualized exercise medicine program. Until then, an exercise medicine prescription is associated with a lower risk of coronary artery disease, coronary heart disease, and peripheral artery disease when compared to less physical activity.

But, here again, the key to carrying out a safe exercise medicine prescription requires (a) teaching the adult the importance of eating and drinking appropriately (e.g., avoid eating 2 hours prior to exercising, drinking plenty of water before, during, and after exercising); (b) warming-up and cooling down correctly by adhering to the "three" good warm-up (i.e., flexibility) exercises; (c) wearing good shoes; and (d) listening to the body by not ignoring aches and pains. Aging adults also need repeated instruction as to exercise frequency, intensity, and time commitment.

The role of exercise physiology in preventive health care is a matter of assessing the adult's physiologic capacity. This can be done with the use of a standard metabolic cart or it can be done as a stepwise process of determining the adult's overall physiologic responses with the use of proven regression equations. What is important here is that the professional that oversees the process is an ASEP Board-Certified Exercise Physiologist and not someone who happens to have an interest in exercising.

What is also important is that the energy cost of physical activities for frail elders with assistive devices (e.g., walkers and wheelchairs) is likely to be much higher than the equations would predict (Singh 2002). Frail adults need individualized attention prior to becoming involved in aerobic training. For example, if standing from a chair is difficult, then resistance training should be prescribed to strengthen the musculoskeletal system before beginning the aerobic training prescription.

## Final Thoughts

Aging is a natural biological reality that is reflected in the mental and physical changes from birth to age 60 years and older, which is known as the elderly period of life. Aside from significant changes in the nervous system and brain function that result in the neurodegenerative conditions like Alzheimer's and Parkinson's diseases, the decrease in muscle mass and strength lead to an increase in risk of fractures and a decrease in quality of life and independence (Faulkner et al. 2007).

To reduce the pandemic of chronic diseases and frailty associated with physical inactivity, physical activity is the treatment of choice. All adults, including the frail elders, who attain a higher level of cardiorespiratory fitness lower their risk of chronic diseases and death. Interestingly, Warburton et al. (2010) reported, "Inactive patients can lower their mortality risk by 10% by simply walking 10 minutes a day." While this point speaks well for the aerobic exercise prescription, it appears that many physicians are not comfortable with prescribing exercise medicine. This point was highlighted by Solmundson et al. (2016), who indicated that 91% of the future physicians want more education and training in how to prescribe exercise medicine.

Here again, the Board-Certified Exercise Physiologist is educated and prepared to write the exercise medicine prescription. This point underscores the importance of the medical community working with ASEP exercise physiologists to prescribe exercise to their patients. Today, perhaps more than ever before, the primary care physician is recognizing that regular exercise is medicine and, if the exercise prescription is done correctly, it has the power to help people live longer, healthier lives. It is for this reason among others that the ASEP exercise physiologist should be recognized as the healthcare professional responsible for writing the aerobic exercise prescription to help avoid the age-associated lowering of the threshold for left ventricular hypertrophy, chronic heart failure, and atrial fibrillation (Lakatta 2002).

Aerobic exercise is a medicine with well-known positive physical benefits, such as (a) the increase in cardiorespiratory fitness among older adults that is linked to an increase in peak cardiac output, stroke volume, ejection fraction, and left ventricular contractility (Schulman et al. 1996); and (b) the decrease in the risk of heart failure, myocardial infarction, and the age-related arterial and cardiac stiffening (Jakovljevic 2018; Lee 2010). Exercise helps to increase more blood flow to brain, thus helping to prevent cognitive decline. It is also clear that aerobic exercise benefits the brain by decreasing the risk of Alzheimer's disease and other dementias (Holmes 2019). Patients who engage in regular exercise are often less depressed, experience fewer falls compared to patients who did not exercise, and have significant gains in functional balance and mobility.

## References

Blair, SN. (2009). Physical Inactivity: The Biggest Public Health Problem of the 21st Century. *British Journal of Sports Medicine*. 43;1–2.

Blair, SN, Kohl, HW, Barlow, CE, et al. (1989). Physical Fitness and All-Cause Mortality: A Perspective Study of Healthy Men and Women. *Journal of the American Medical Association*. 262(17);2395–2401.

Boone, T. (2014). *Introduction to Exercise Physiology*. Burlington, MA: Jones & Bartlett Publishers.

Boone, T. (2016). *ASEP's Exercise Medicine Text for Exercise Physiologists*. Sharjah, UAE: Bentham Science Publishing.

Booth, FW, Laye, MJ, Roberts, MD. (2011). Lifetime Sedentary Living Accelerates Some Aspects of Secondary Aging. *Journal of Applied Physiology*. 111(5);1497–1504.

Ciolac, EG. (2013). Exercise Training as a Preventive Tool for Age-Related Disorders: A Brief Review. *Clinics*. 68(5);710–717.

Faulkner, JA, Larkin, LM, Claflin, DR, Brooks, SV. (2007). Age-Related Changes in the Structure and Function of the Skeletal Muscles. *Clinical and Experimental Pharmacology and Physiology*. 34(11); 1091–1096.

Holmes, B. (2019). The Workout Drug. *Knowable Magazine* [Online]. www. knowablemagazine.org/ article/health-disease/2019/exercise-as-medicine

Jakovljevic, DG. (2018). Physical Activity and Cardiovascular Aging: Physiological and Molecular Insights. *Experimental Gerontology*. 109;67–74.

Lakatta, EG. (2002). Age-Associated Cardiovascular Changes in Health: Impact on Cardiovascular Disease in Older Persons. *Heart Failure Review*. 7(1);29–49.

Lee, IM. (2010). Physical Activity and Cardiac Protection. *Current Sports Medicine Reports*. 9;214–219.

Lee, IM, Shiroma, EJ, Lobelo F, et al. (2012). Lancet Physical Activity Series Working group. Effects of Physical Inactivity on Major Non-Communicable Diseases Worldwide: An Analysis of Burden of Disease and Life Expectancy. *Lancet*. 380;219–229.

Naci, H, Ioannidis, JP. (2015). Comparative Effectiveness of Exercise and Drug Interventions on Mortality Outcomes: Meta-Epidemiological Study. *British Journal of Sports Medicine*. 49;1414–1422.

Saltin, B, Blomqvist, G, Mitchell, JH, Johnson, RL, Jr., Wildenthal, K, Chapman, CB. (1968). Response to Exercise After Bed Rest and After Training. *Circulation*. 38(5);VIII–VII78.

Schuch, FP, Vancammpfort D, Firth J, et al. (2018). Physical Activity and Incident Depression: A Meta-Analysis of Prospective Cohort Studies. *American Journal of Psychiatry*. 175;631–648.

Schulman, S, Fleg, JL, Goldberg, AP, et al. (1996). Continuum of Cardiovascular Performance Across a Broad Range of Fitness Levels in Healthy Older Men. *Circulation*. 94;359–367.

Singh, MAF. (2002). Exercise Comes of Age: Rationale and Recommendations for a Geriatric Exercise Prescription. *Journal of Gerontology: Medical Sciences*. 57A(5); M262–M282.

Solmundson, K, Koehle, M, McKenzie, D. (2016). Are We Adequately Preparing the Next Generation of Physicians to Prescribe Exercise as Prevention and Treatment? Residents Express the Desire for More Training in Exercise Prescription. *Canadian Medical Education Journal*. 7;e79–e96.

Struthers, R, Erasmus, P, Holmes, K, et al. (2008). Assessing Fitness for Surgery: A Comparison of Questionnaire, Incremental Shuttle Walk, and Cardiopulmonary Exercise Testing in General Surgical Patients. *British Journal of Anaesthesia*. 101(6);774–780.

Thompson, WR, Joy, E, Jaworski, CA, et al. (2020). Exercise Is Medicine. *American Journal of Lifestyle Medicine*. 1–13 [Online]. https://journals.sagepub.com/doi/pdf/10.1177/1559827620912 192

Warburton, DE, Charlesworth, S, Ivey, A, et al. (2010). A Systematic Review of the Evidence for Canada's Physical Activity Guidelines for Adults. *International Journal of Behavioral Nutrition and Physical Activity*. 7(1);1–220.

# PART IV
# Exercise Medicine Professionals

# 12

# EXERCISE PHYSIOLOGISTS ARE HEALTHCARE PROFESSIONALS

Exercise medicine is the logical step to cutting the cost of treating illness and improving quality of life. Exercise is medicine, and when properly prescribed it is better than the equivalent of a bottle of prescription pills. Moreover, it is becoming increasingly clear among healthcare professionals that the so-called exercise pill is not the answer in treating chronic diseases. The work of an exercise physiologist in prescribing regular exercise confers short- and long-term health benefits.

Fortunately, the leaders of the American Society of Exercise Physiologists (ASEP) understood this point of view years ago. That is part of the reason they founded the organization, but they didn't stop there. They created the first-ever professional definition of an exercise physiologist, a code of ethics to guide the exercise physiologist's professional standards of practice, academic accreditation guidelines for college programs, and board certification for exercise physiologists. The ASEP organization is now 25 years old, and the leadership continues to do what is necessary to promote exercise physiologists as healthcare professionals.

The network of Exercise Physiologists who are Board-Certified represents a collective group of professionals with the academic and hands-on laboratory skills to safely and effectively prescribe the medicine of exercise in the prevention and treatment of ill-health and improve the quality of life of individuals living with chronic disease. After all, it is abundantly clear that exercise changes the way our bodies work at the molecular level. Think about it for a moment. Exercise medicine burns off the excess fat, protects us from chronic diseases, builds the musculoskeletal system, and overall helps us be happier people (Boone 2014a).

## Medicine in the Form of Exercise

Exercise medicine is the prescriptive drug for protecting us against hypertension, cardiovascular disease, type 2 diabetes, certain types of cancer, and much more! Yes, "medicine" in the form of walking for 30 to 50 min 3 times·wk$^{-1}$ can promote weight loss, a decrease in blood pressure and cholesterol, and bring about a reduction in the body's inflammatory state, and much more (Boone 2016). The improvement in overall fitness of the mind and body is real and far-reaching. Yes, the medical community will no doubt get involved in talking about the

DOI: 10.4324/9781003119920-16

benefits of exercise, but it isn't likely that medical doctors are going to move too far from the prescription of pills in the usual containers Americans pay for on a regular basis.

This is true even though the prescription of exercise medicine is better for all of us than the usual over-the-counter pills. How many prescription drugs can one person take for this and that disease and the predisposition to other diseases? The answer is an average of about six different pills a day. Yet regular exercise for 30 $min \cdot d^{-1}$ every day of the week or 50 $min \cdot d^{-1}$ 3 $times \cdot wk^{-1}$ improves body function, reduces anxiety, depression, and the decline in cognitive function.

The bottom line should not be hard to grasp, especially given that exercise medicine improves the quality of life while adding years to your life. Imagine waking up and going for a walk instead of taking six or more pills. Which is better, the pills or the exercise medicine, which is likely to be more effective than the prescription drugs and also without negative side effects as well. Imagine, on one hand exercise and on the other hand a higher risk of chronic disease. Which do you want? Or, aerobic exercise just 15 $min \cdot d^{-1}$ of moderate-intensity exercise (such as a brisk walk) or the daily challenges associated with a progressive cognitive impairment with aging? What about resistance exercise training that builds lean muscle mass and strength or continues to suffer from sarcopenia and progressive aging? Would you rather exercise medicine on a regular basic with the help of a qualified exercise physiology healthcare professional or the loss of range of motion (flexibility) of the skeletal muscles with an increase in the risk of falls?

Life should be about improving mind and body function with aging, not about losing function or otherwise life becomes difficult to tolerate. Board-Certified Exercise Physiologists understand this point very well. That is why they use the **ASEP's Exercise Medicine Text for Exercise Physiologists** (Boone 2016) when providing health care to patients (or clients) who are predisposed to or have one or more chronic diseases. They understand that exercise medicine helps with the issues their patients and families care about, that is, mental and physical functioning, independence, and quality of life. Exercise medicine is powerfully protective of life by decreasing blood fats (LDL and triglycerides) that contribute to clogged arteries. It helps in raising HDL cholesterol and decreasing high blood sugar while improving insulin sensitivity that indicates a lower likelihood of developing diabetes and other diseases and disorders.

---

**BOX 12.1   AGING PRESENTS AN ARRAY OF DISEASES AND DISORDERS.**

From 2010 to 2030, an additional 27 million people will have hypertension, 8 million will have coronary heart disease, 4 million will have stroke, and 3 million will have heart failure due to the rapid accumulation of elders.

—Heidenreich et al. (2011). Forecasting the Future of Cardiovascular Disease in the United States: A Policy Statement from the American Heart Association. *Circulation.* 123;933–944.

---

Also, in terms of slowing the aging process that is linked to the decrease in the energy-generating capacity of the mitochondria, exercise medicine helps the cells to produce more RNA copies of genes coding for mitochondrial proteins and proteins responsible for lean muscle development.

## The Problem

Although society is full of obesity and physical inactivity, people of all ages will do just about anything to avoid exercising. Do they understand the long-term effects of chronic inactivity? The short answer is "yes"—at least at a certain level they know that regular exercise (i.e., exercise medicine) is necessary to optimize health and well-being. Does that mean they are going to jump up from the couch and go for a walk in their neighborhood? No, and yet just 150 min·wk$^{-1}$ would help keep them healthy. So, what is the problem? What is keeping billions of people from acting in their own best interest? No doubt the lack of desire to engage in exercise medicine is much more complex than we think.

Lieberman (2015) thinks the lack of exercise is a function of our evolutionary history. He maintains that the most effective way to encourage people to exercise is to make exercise more enjoyable. Whether it is in the workplace, at school, or in the community where people live, when people look forward to having fun while exercising, they are more likely to participate and, perhaps, do so on a regular basis. He also concludes that society should do what it can to restore the need to be active throughout our environment. So, in a nutshell, with the increase in technology that influences essentially all aspects of our lives, the problem (it seems to me) is one of "having fun" or at least "contemplating positive and relaxing thoughts" while exercising. If it is not fun and/or relaxing, why do it? If it is somewhat fun and perceived as necessary, maybe there is the possibility of engaging in regular exercise. Either way, the problem of inactivity and early death and/or disability from chronic diseases raises the question, is it worth it even if it isn't that much fun? The answer is "yes" if you want to live a longer and healthier life.

With regard to the "fun" idea, people do many different things to experience a positive feeling of happiness. It might be watching a football game or track event on TV or even reading a book. Not everyone and in fact not many people engage in acts of physical strength and endurance (i.e., lifting weights and/or running distances). You might say the problem is simply that the majority of the people, regardless of age and/or sex, are not interested in being physically active as in exercising on a regular basis. But an additional part of the problem is that the majority of the people in the United States must get over the idea that they can avoid their responsibility in taking care of their mind and body. The bottom line is that they can't turn a blind eye or a deaf ear to the importance of regular exercise. Thus, part of the role of the ASEP Board-Certified Exercise Physiologist is to talk about exercise medicine and its role in maintaining and/or enhancing physical fitness and general health and well-being.

## Looking Ahead: Exercise Medicine

Several facts about exercise medicine are worth highlighting over and over. There are many published research papers indicating that exercise improves the mind by decreasing anxiety and promoting a positive mood, improves sex, reduces breast cancer after menopause, and decreases the habit of consuming too many calories. For some individuals, the exercise can be the "light" type, for others, the "moderate" type, and still for others, the "vigorous" type. Regardless of the intensity, however, the key is regular participation in one of the three (i.e., walking, for example, vs. running), and then the exerciser can expect to experience a decrease in the risk of high blood pressure, diabetes, and cholesterol, among other positive outcomes.

---

## BOX 12.2 EXERCISE, FRAILTY, AND SARCOPENIA IN THE AGING POPULATION.

"Increased physical activity could provide a nonpharmacological preventive approach to augmenting patient quality of life and function, and could conceivably improve the ability to tolerate pharmacological and interventional treatment of CV conditions, hence improving CV outcomes."

—Paneni, F, Canestro, CD, Libby, P, et al. (2017). The Aging Cardiovascular System: Understanding it at the Cellular and Clinical Levels. *Journal of the American College of Cardiology.* 69(15);1952–1967.

---

The elderly frail adult can also expect to improve the body's consumption of oxygen (i.e., $VO_2$), which is used in the mitochondria within the muscle cells to produce adenosine triphosphate (ATP) (i.e., energy) for muscle contraction. In this case, light to moderate exercise is more likely to be "aerobic" exercise versus the vigorous type that may compromise the availability of oxygen at the cell level to produce energy sufficient to keep the muscles working without a high level of fatigue. Looking ahead, the question is this for the patient and client. "Are you interested in your health and well-being to the point of walking around the block every night after eating supper?" Before he or she answers, they should also think about the fact that exercise decreases stress, feelings of anxiety, and symptoms of depression.

Aerobic exercise medicine results in stronger muscles, stronger heart, decreased blood pressure, improved circulatory response throughout the body, increased red blood cells that improve the transport of oxygen to the muscles, improved mental health and sleep quality with a reduction in migraine symptoms, decreased risk of heart disease and other cardiovascular problems, increased bone growth and decreased risk of osteoporosis, increased blood flow to the muscles, increase in skeletal muscular stamina, and an increase in cardiovascular endurance. As to anaerobic exercise (which is still exercise medicine), the benefits are equally important. They are increased expenditure of energy that helps to control the bodyweight along with stronger muscles, bones, and joints (Nordqvist 2017).

The long and short of it is that the ASEP organization created the necessary professional credentials to move exercise physiology forward as a healthcare profession. The leadership emphasizes quality over profit, an updated and accredited curriculum and laboratory facilities, and Board Certification to distinguish the ASEP exercise physiologist from graduates and/or membership of other programs and/or organizations. They have connected regular exercise, prevention, and public health concerns (particularly as they relate to lifestyle-mediated chronic diseases).

There is also strong evidence that exercise medicine improves the pathogenesis and symptoms of coronary heart disease, chronic heart failure, hypertension, obesity, dyslipidemia, intermittent claudication, insulin resistance, and type 2 diabetes mellitus (Pedersen & Saltin 2006). There is excellent research supporting exercise medicine as a healthcare intervention for osteoporosis, and the symptoms of chronic obstructive pulmonary disease, fibromyalgia, mental depression, and osteoarthritis. With the professional guidance, there is a very serious healthcare opportunity to prevent certain chronic non–communicable diseases better than the traditional medical use of prescriptive drugs.

## Exercise Medicine and the Curriculum

Yes, up to this point, the content has been about benefits and the push for exercise medicine. Unfortunately, there are pieces of the puzzle that are yet to be updated. In particular, across the United States, the academic institutions, the degree plans, and the college graduates' pursuit of a career in exercise medicine are also up in the air. The undergraduate degree in exercise physiology is either an ASEP accredited degree or it is one of a dozen or more degree programs with different degree titles, such as exercise science, sports science, kinesiology, human performance, and others. Many of these degree programs are a transition in title with little change in the original curriculum of the health and physical education degree.

The ASEP leaders characterize the non-ASEP accredited exercise physiology degree programs as being in a state of disarray due primarily to the lack of a specific intended purpose in mind. That is, the degree programs do not provide the students access to a credible career as the exercise physiology degree does after college. In fact, the lack of discussion regarding career opportunities in the academic departments is so bad that the advisors simply tell the students to make application for graduate school (such as it is time to apply to physical therapy or nursing). Why? The short answer is because the faculty members have done very little to prepare the college graduates to move into a specific career-driven field of professional work.

Sad to say, but the professors are primarily interested in doing research, publishing papers, getting access to grants, and attending national meetings. Teaching is of little interest in many academic settings. The professors have been emphasizing research over quality teaching for decades and, frankly, they have no desire to contemplate the differences between the exercise science degree and the exercise physiology degree. Many may even believe that a minor in exercise physiology with a major in kinesiology allows them to refer to their students as exercise physiologists! Such thinking is sad and disappointing, and it must change along with the inadequate curricula throughout the different academic programs (Boone 2001, 2005, 2006, 2009, 2014b).

For all of its assumed benefits, the college degree that is not designed with a credible career purpose in mind is a meaningless degree program. There is an urgent need for the faculty of these related degree programs to dedicate time to rethinking degree titles and the respective curricula. They need to equip their students with the right laboratory skills and healthcare knowledge and confidence to promote exercise medicine as a viable career option after college. Students need information about how to start an exercise medicine clinic and the actual specifics and practice of working with and counseling patients and clients (Boone 2012). The students' lack of behavioral counseling knowledge, lifestyle medicine training, and/or skills in the business of starting an exercise medicine healthcare business is hugely problematic. The ASEP leadership has been talking and writing about these concerns for years.

Yet little to almost no serious change in the academic infrastructure has taken place. The present situation is a far cry from the expected behavior of men and women who have the doctorate degree. In fact, it is remarkable that parents are still sending their children to college. Moreover, it is worth asking the following question: Given the present situation, why not just get a generic personal trainer certification from one of the 300 different groups who will be more than happy to take your money? An advantage of the ASEP accredited exercise physiology degree is that the students at graduation are prepared to demonstrate proficiency in exercise medicine assessment, exercise prescription and implementation, counseling for a better mind, and the specifics of improving body health and fitness.

## Final Thoughts

It is clear from the scientific papers that regular exercise prevents chronic diseases, which lowers the rate of mortality throughout the world. Compared to active individuals, sedentary patients' medical costs attributed to inactivity is in the billions of dollars. Inactivity will break the bank for healthcare spending (Sallis 2009). Such a statement would seem to open the eyes of the medical community, but it hasn't. Little is being done by the medical profession to bring about an increase in physical activity throughout the United States. Yet exercise is medicine (or more to the point); exercise medicine should be prescribed by exercise medicine professionals, who are in fact ASEP Board-Certified Exercise Physiologists. There should be a merging of the different academic degrees that have a similarity to the exercise physiology degree so that the college graduates of ASEP accredited exercise physiology academic institution can be in a better position to help society improve the health of individuals young and old. Exercise physiology professors in the academic institutions of exercise science, kinesiology, or human performance should become more active in the change process promoted by ASEP. In fact, it is imperative that the students understand the differences in the academic degree programs and their role ultimately in health care to reduce the risk associated with sedentary living while at the same time increase credible career opportunities for their students throughout the United States.

## References

Boone, T. (2001). *Professional Development of Exercise Physiology*. Lewiston, NY: The Edwin Mellen Press.

Boone, T. (2005). *Exercise Physiology: Professional Issues, Organizational Concerns, and Ethical Trends*. Lewiston, NY: The Edwin Mellen Press.

Boone, T. (2006). *Exercise Physiology as a Career: A Guide and Sourcebook*. Lewiston, NY: The Edwin Mellen Press.

Boone, T. (2009). *The Professionalization of Exercise Physiology: Certification, Accreditation, and Standards of Practice of the American Society of Exercise Physiologists (ASEP)*. Lewiston, NY: The Edwin Mellen Press.

Boone, T. (2012). *The Business of Exercise Physiology: Thinking Like an Entrepreneur*. Lewiston, NY: The Edwin Mellen Press.

Boone, T. (2014a). *Introduction to Exercise Physiology*. Burlington, MA: Jones & Bartlett Publishing.

Boone, T. (2014b). *Promoting Professionalism in Exercise Physiology: Visions, Challenges, and Opportunities*. Lewiston, NY: The Edwin Mellen Press.

Boone, T. (2016). *ASEP's Exercise Medicine Text for Exercise Physiologists*. Sharjah, UAE: Bentham Science Publishers.

Heidenreich, PA, Trogdon JG, Khavyou OA, et al. (2011). Forecasting the Future of Cardiovascular Disease in the United States: A Policy Statement from the American Heart Association, *Circulation*. 123;933–944.

Lieberman, DE. (2015). Is Exercise Really Medicine? An Evolutionary Perspective. *Current Sports Medicine Reports*. 14(4);313–319.

Nordqvist, C. (2017). Exercise: Health Benefits, Types, How It Works. *Medical News Today* [Online]. www.medicalnewstoday.com/articles/153390.php.

Paneni, F, Canestro, CD, Libby, P, et al. (2017). The Aging Cardiovascular System: Understanding It at the Cellular and Clinical Levels. *Journal of the American College of Cardiology.* 69(15);1952–1967.

Pedersen, BK, Saltin, B. (2006). Evidence for Prescribing Exercise as Therapy in Chronic Disease. *Scandinavian Journal of Medicine & Science in Sports.* 16(1);3–63.

Sallis, R.E. (2009). Exercise Is Medicine and Physicians Need to Prescribe It! *British Journal of Sports Medicine.* 43(1);3–4.

# 13

# A CALL TO ACTION FOR EXERCISE PHYSIOLOGISTS

The research is clear that regular exercise is a powerful medicine for both the prevention and treatment of chronic diseases (Boone 2016b). Moreover, it is helpful in dealing with obesity and its negative effects on health and wellness. Individuals who do not exercise on a regular basis are less active and are likely to live an unhealthy lifestyle. The association between being physically inactive and living with a chronic disease exists in all individuals regardless of age and gender (Booth 2012).

Unfortunately, however, the inactive and sedentary lifestyle is so common that many people fail to acknowledge it as a risk factor for early disease and/or death. Why this is the case is a mystery. On one hand, it is simply easier and more direct to deal with an obvious disease by prescribing a drug while, on the other hand, speaking to a client or patient about his or her behaviors that correlate with quality of health isn't always easy to do.

Only a small percent of people react in a positive way to talking about the importance of starting an exercise program, stopping smoking, and monitoring one's diet and losing weight. Yet the question: Why isn't exercise medicine, health, and fitness a topic of interest among adults in particular? Also, equally interesting with all the talk among certain researchers, but not among the majority of the academic types is the little-discussed steps to ensure that the students of exercise physiology are involved in an intensive study of the dangers of inactivity. After all, exercise medicine can save lives.

---

**BOX 13.1   EXERCISE MEDICINE.**

Exercise physiologists have known for decades that exercise is medicine. The scientific evidence is clear. Regular exercise helps to prevent chronic disease and premature death. Exercise physiologists are "the" healthcare providers of exercise medicine.

---

Specifically, why aren't the academic programs in the Departments of Exercise Physiology accredited by the **American Society of Exercise Physiologists**? Why aren't the students sitting for the ASEP Board Certification? This does not make sense, given ASEP's emphasis

DOI: 10.4324/9781003119920-17

on the "Exercise Physiologist Certification" and exercise medicine. Similarly, why aren't the physicians referring their patients who are either inactive or have recognized chronic disease to the ASEP exercise physiologists?

Considering that ASEP is the first profession-specific organization of exercise physiologists in the United States with an emphasis on accreditation, certification, and exercise medicine, it seems logical to reach out to the leadership to build a bridge between ASEP and the healthcare industry. Moreover, it is time that ASEP Board-Certified Exercise Physiologists are recognized as credible healthcare professionals who have the education and laboratory training to prescribe exercise medicine (ASEP 2019a).

So why has the academic community neglected updating exercise science major to the exercise physiology major as "the" recognized major for prescribing exercise medicine? The answer to that question is very complex, but I suspect it is just a matter of time and it is easier to keep the academic system the way it has been for decades rather than dealing with the accreditation issues and concerns. The other issue is the obvious lack of support from the related academic majors.

For example, where is it that exercise science, kinesiology, sports science, and human performance are stepping up to the plate of change? They, too, could update their academic curriculum and degree title to exercise physiology and thousands of students would benefit. However, it is clear that the change process is very slow. In addition, the deans, department chairs, and faculty seem to be transferring the responsibility for credible career opportunities away from them and onto the students. As long as the college professors continue to avoid responsibility for promoting the work of the American Society of Exercise Physiologists on behalf of accreditation and exercise medicine, it is unlikely we will see a big increase in ASEP accredited programs in the next year.

Yet it makes sense that exercise physiologists should lead the effort in promoting exercise medicine for individuals of all ages and gender. Exercise physiologists have the expertise in helping clients and patients initiate and continue with an exercise medicine prescription (Box 13.2). It is also clear that these healthcare professionals can have their greatest influence on the educational points of exercise medicine by explaining the physiology that undergirds the prescription for exercise. In addition, the ASEP leadership should engage as many exercise physiology entrepreneurs in the public sector as an essential part of getting different communities of individuals involved in at least 150 $min \cdot wk^{-1}$ of regular exercise to stay fit and healthy.

---

**BOX 13.2   EXERCISE PHYSIOLOGY IS THE ESSENCE OF EXERCISE MEDICINE.**

Exercise physiologists have an important responsibility to be the glue that keeps exercise medicine at the very center of its professional development. After all, exercise medicine is real. It has the power to prevent diseases, cut American spending of >3 trillion on health care every year, and increase Americans' average life expectancy.

---

## Physiology of the Exercise Physiologist's Practice

Recently, a friend asked the following question: Will you describe what you mean by educating the students of exercise physiology about the benefits of exercise medicine? I said, Yes, I will be glad to. But please understand the process of doing so does not happen overnight. I have always believed that it would be a great idea to talk about the benefits of regular exercise while being physically active with my students versus just in the classroom. The more students know the more likely they are to make the right decisions about exercise and how it brings about an increase in health and well-being, and the more likely they will be able to help their clients stay with an individualized exercise medicine program. That is why it is necessary to go into some detail about the science of exercise. Students need to know about the knowledge and integrity that comes from understanding the physiological responses and the long-term adaptations. This can be done as part of the exercise medicine prescription that is taught in the students' exercise physiology courses and associated laboratory experiences.

Understandably, there is much more to this process of educating students. But, for now, I hope that my response to the question as well as the following content will help the reader appreciate a few of the basic points important to the physiology of exercise, which should help to motivate the students to live an active lifestyle. After all, as future exercise physiologists versus being physically inactive and sedentary, they have a major responsibility to their clients as well as their own future financial well-being. Hence, without question, the research into the physiology of exercise medicine shows that regular exercise is both an attitude and a physical engagement in a new way of thinking and living.

Ultimately, however, it is obvious that the majority of adults are resistant to being active, decreasing their body fat, and acquiring a positive state of mind about exercise. Whereas a new outlook on life would mean a longer life with less disease and disability, of course it comes about with dedication, discipline, and a positive state of mind. So, in a nutshell, why wouldn't a college graduate get out of the chair and get with an exercise program? Why wouldn't his father, brother, wife, friend, or the young boy across the street want to be healthy, strong, and more in control? Interestingly, that is the question, isn't it? Thus, the point of what I am sharing is that knowing why we need to exercise versus exercise simply for the sake of doing so should help make a difference in a person's commitment to a longer and healthier life (Boone 2013, 2018).

To begin this process of change while reading the following information about the physiologic responses to regular exercise and adaptations, keep in mind that I am describing these responses as part of the philosophy that undergirds the exercise medicine lifestyle. Also, I understand that the students' future clients aren't likely to understand 5% of what will be presented in the following pages. Please keep in that most everything really important begins with the first few steps and the first words of a different path, that is, a different way to think about exercise and life. Without making such an effort, nothing will change and chronic diseases, frailty and disability, and early death will continue to increase throughout the world in big cities and small towns throughout the United States. This isn't good. We must individually and collectively accept the responsibility for not giving in to society's status quo. We must change how we live, and the change process begins with educating individuals of all ages and genders and race about the significance of exercise medicine in healing the mind and body and to sustain and empower life.

To open the door of exercise physiology as exercise medicine professionals is to speak to what is critical, such as the air we breathe. While it is understandable that the body needs oxygen ($O_2$) to produce energy for muscle contraction to be more physically productive, oftentimes we fail to appreciate that with each breath the body needs to get rid of carbon dioxide ($CO_2$) to maintain an acid–base balance. Both are done through the response of the respiratory and cardiovascular systems. At rest, a client who weighs 70 kg (154 lbs) will consume an average volume of oxygen ($VO_2$) equal to approximately 250 mL·min⁻¹. The transition from rest to walking causes the lungs to work harder by breathing more frequently and deeper per breath per minute. The first is referred to as frequency of breaths (Fb), and the second is called tidal volume ($T_V$), which is the volume of air breathed in with each breath. Hence, an increase in Fb from 12 to 20 breaths·min⁻¹ and a Tv change from 500 mL to 1000 mL·breath⁻¹ increases the volume of oxygen inhaled and $CO_2$ exhaled, which is known as expired ventilation ($V_E$, L·min⁻¹) (Boone 2013, 2018).

The $VO_2$ response is a function of how much $O_2$ is needed at the cellular level to produce energy in the form of ATP (i.e., adenosine triphosphate) that is used by the muscles to contract and bring about movement (such as walking). With the increase in response of the lungs to exercise, the work of the myocardium (i.e., heart) is increased to make sure there is an increase in $O_2$ at the peripheral tissues throughout the body. This is done by increasing heart rate (HR) and stroke volume (SV, which is the volume of blood ejected from the ventricles with each ventricular contraction or heartbeat). At rest, SV is ~70 mL·beat⁻¹ ejected from each ventricle. Hence, the left ventricle pumps ~70 mL of blood carrying $O_2$ with each contraction. The blood enters the aorta to find its way via a multitude of large to smaller arteries in the peripheral tissues (i.e., muscles in particular), while 70 mL of blood from the right ventricle is loaded with a higher carbon dioxide ($CO_2$) content that is pumped to the lungs (Boone 2013, 2018).

Hence, given an average resting HR of 70 beats·min⁻¹ and an average SV of 70 mL, the volume of blood ejected from the heart is ~5,000 mL·min⁻¹ or 5 L·min⁻¹, which is consistent with the average $VO_2$ at rest of .25 L·min⁻¹. The $O_2$ in the lungs diffuses into the blood to be carried by hemoglobin (Hb) to form oxyhemoglobin ($HbO_2$) that goes to the heart. From the heart (specifically, the left ventricle), the $O_2$ in the blood is pumped to the muscle tissues throughout the body. The 1-min ejection of blood from the left ventricle to the muscles is referred to as cardiac output (Q), which is equal to the product of HR and SV.

At rest, the volume of $O_2$ pumped by the left ventricle to the muscles by the 5 L·min⁻¹ Q is increased with the transition from rest to exercise because the muscles need more $O_2$ to contract more frequently per minute of exercise. The increase in Q occurs by way of an automatic increase in HR due to the role of the sympathetic nervous system (SNS), which is a division of the autonomic nervous system. The SNS also increases ventricular contractility that results in a larger SV. The latter response is important because it helps to eject more blood from the ventricles during each contraction. If HR is increased to 130 beats·min⁻¹ and SV is increased to 95 mL·bt⁻¹ from rest to moderate-intensity exercise, Q would be 12,350 mL·min⁻¹ or 12.35 L·min⁻¹ (Boone 2013, 2018).

The increase in Q provides more $O_2$ to the muscles by way of what is known as arteriovenous oxygen difference (a-v$O_2$ diff), which is the difference between the oxygen content of the arterial blood to the muscles and the venous blood leaving the muscles to return to the heart and then to the lungs. The a-v$O_2$ diff is an indication of how much oxygen is removed from the arterial blood in the capillaries as the blood circulates throughout the body. At rest, the left ventricle generally pumps 20 mL of $O_2$ per 100 mL of blood or 20 mL·dL⁻¹ with a venous $O_2$ difference of 15 mL of $O_2$ per 100 mL of blood (15 mL·dL⁻¹). Thus, at rest it becomes apparent that the muscles consume 5 mL·dL⁻¹ of blood. This difference at rest indicates that 25% of the $O_2$ is removed from each 100 mL of blood as the blood passes through the tissues. The oxygen is used in the electron transport system within the mitochondria of the muscle cells to provide energy in the form of ATP for muscle contraction and other cellular needs (Boone 2013, 2018).

During exercise, the muscles need more energy, which is accomplished by increasing the dissociation of $O_2$ from the Hb in the blood at the cell level. Hence, the a-v$O_2$ diff is expected to increase from the 5 mL·dL$^{-1}$ of blood to 10 or 15 mL·dL$^{-1}$ (depending on the intensity of the exercise). The increase is necessary to supply the $O_2$ that is needed to produce more ATP to allow for a greater increase in muscle contraction. Again, this means there is less $O_2$ in the venous blood leaving the muscles, which returns to the heart and ultimately to the lungs. In the lungs, the $CO_2$ in the venous blood goes into the lungs to be exhaled. At the same time, the increase in HR and SV produces a larger Q that continues to deliver a full volume of $O_2$ per 100 mL to the tissues. As a result, the resting $VO_2$ increases to match the muscular workload, which may be (as an example) a submaximal exercise $VO_2$ of 1,500 mL·min$^{-1}$ (or 1.5 L·min$^{-1}$) at 600 kpm·min$^{-1}$ on a bicycle ergometer. This means the myocardium must get the first supply of rich oxygenated blood ejected from the left ventricle via the coronary arteries to the upper and lower chambers of the heart. The continuous blood flow to the different muscular structures of the heart is the means by which the heart continues to work in supplying blood to all the muscular and other tissues throughout the body (Boone 2013, 2018). At this point, it is beginning to make sense to the client that the integrity of the lungs and the heart is critical to supplying the body (especially the muscles during exercise) with the $O_2$ from the air we breathe to the peripheral tissues. As the blood from the right ventricle goes to the lungs, it interfaces with the pulmonary capillaries. The higher pressure of $O_2$ in the lungs and the pulmonary capillaries versus the venous blood drives the $O_2$ from the lungs into the blood. The blood leaving the lungs is saturated with $O_2$ to be dispersed throughout the body. Ultimately, the functional integrity of the lungs and the heart is matched by the metabolic needs of the peripheral tissues. Gradually, the client will come to understand that $VO_2$ is the product of Q (HR × SV) and a-v$O_2$ diff (i.e., the $O_2$ that is delivered by the heart and the $O_2$ that is used by the peripheral cells) (Boone 2013, 2018).

While clients do not need to be treated as students in an exercise physiology course, it is reasonable to think they would be more motivated to exercise if they knew some of the information just presented. Just think, after age 25 or so, $VO_2$ decreases 9% to 15% per year. Why, because age (or rather lack of regular exercise) is associated with the decrease in Q and a-v$O_2$ diff. Aging is in a sense the opposite of regular exercise. Without exercise, the body ages and with aging there is the decrease in structure and function of the body parts. Also, please appreciate that this brief assessment of the client's physiology is just #1 out of at least 50 bits of information (Boone 2016b) that could be the key to helping a person to stay with the exercise medicine prescription (Boone 2013, 2018).

Myocardial oxygen uptake ($MVO_2$) is determined by the Board-Certified Exercise Physiologist through the use of a regression formula, such as [$MVO_2$ = .14 (HR × SBP × .01) − 6.3]. The product of HR and systolic blood pressure (SBP) is called double product (DP). It is a linear relation between $MVO_2$ and coronary blood flow. During exercise, HR increases linearly with workload and $VO_2$. Systolic blood pressure rises with increased work as a result of the increase in Q, while diastolic blood pressure usually remains the same or decreases somewhat. Failure of SBP to rise with exercise can be the result of aortic outflow obstruction, left ventricular dysfunction, or myocardial ischemia. Changes in blood pressure may also reflect peripheral vascular resistance, given that systemic vascular resistance (SVR) equals mean arterial pressure (MAP) divided by Q. Since Q is expected to increase with progressive increments in exercise work and MAP usually changes very little, then SVR is expected to decrease with exercise (Boone 2016b).

## Measurement and Examination

Exercise physiology **measurement and examination** includes (a) giving a health history questionnaire, a disease-specific or disorder-specific laboratory evaluation that includes analysis of the musculoskeletal system and/or cardiorespiratory system using standard laboratory equipment, exercise tests protocols, exercise programs, and risk factor modification and/or measurements to assist in evaluating the client's overt and/or objective responses, signs, and/or symptoms for cardiorespiratory fitness of individuals who are apparently healthy or who have a chronic disease including, but are not limited to, tests that measure body composition, range of motion (flexibility), muscle strength, endurance, work, and power; (b) tests that assist in the analysis of the central and peripheral components of oxygen consumption and energy expenditure; (c) tests of pulmonary function, and exercise prescription for cardiorespiratory fitness training of individuals with metabolic disorders that include, but not limited to, issues and/or deficiencies of the cardiovascular system, diabetes, lipid disorders, hypertension, cancer, cystic fibrosis, chronic obstructive and restrictive pulmonary diseases, arthritis, organ transplant, peripheral vascular disease, and obesity; and (d) treadmill or other ergometer test protocols in conjunction with exercise electrocardiography (ECG) to identify the HR and ECG issues at rest and during submaximal and maximal (graded) exercise programs in addition to specific contraindications for continuing exercise (ASEP 2019b).

## Instruction

Exercise physiology **instruction** includes providing educational, consultative, or other advisory services for the purpose of helping the public with issues and concerns regarding fundamental and scientific information about mind–body health and fitness. **Instruction** pertains to matters that are believed to develop and/or maintain the subject's health, fitness, and rehabilitation. It includes but may not be limited to (a) acute physiological responses to exercise; (b) chronic physiological adaptations to training; (c) designing resistance training programs; (d) measuring energy expenditure at rest and during different types of exercise; (e) hormonal regulation and/or metabolic adaptations to aerobic and anaerobic training; (f) cardiorespiratory regulation and adaptation during exercise; (g) thermal regulation during exercise; (h) exercising at altitude, underwater, and in space; (i) optimizing sports training through the use of ergogenic aids and better nutrition; (j) appropriate body composition and optimal bodyweight and the role each plays in diabetes and physical activity; (k) growth and development of young athletes, aging, and gender issues; (l) preventing cardiovascular disease through exercise; (m) biomechanical aspects of posture and sports and the physiological assessment of human movement; (n) stress testing protocols for athletes and special populations; (o) resting and exercise electrocardiography changes; (p) biobehavioral techniques for reducing stress while increasing running economy; and (q) biochemistry of nutrition and exercise.

## Analysis and Treatment

Exercise physiology **analysis** and **treatment** includes performing laboratory tests, with specific expectations for treatment measures and activities. This may include but is not limited to (a) a range of motion (flexibility) exercises; (b) muscle strength and muscle endurance exercises; (c) lean muscle tissue-fat analysis; (d) musculoskeletal and/or postural exercises; (e) sports nutrition programs; (f) sports biomechanics instructions for the enhancement of sports- or occupational-related skills; (g) stress management exercises; (h) sports training and the development programs; (i) cardiac and pulmonary rehabilitation (including, but not limited to, the development of such programs, supervising testing, development of exercise prescription, and other functions of educating and counseling of athletes, clients, and patients); and (j) exercise physiology instruction that pertains to all forms of exercise medicine programs, sports training, and athletics (ASEP 2019a).

## Final Thoughts

Physical activity can be designed as physical exercise, which can be prescribed as exercise medicine by an ASEP Board-Certified Exercise Physiologist to decrease risk factors linked to chronic diseases and disabilities. Why then aren't more adults exercising and seeking out the guidance of an exercise physiologist? The short answer is that it requires a state of mind that is different from the present way of thinking. Most people simply do not have the discipline to exercise even though they may understand it is necessary. It is easier to play on the computer or watch a football game on TV and consume calories from redundant eating. When it does click that their blood pressure is elevated or that they have gained another 10 lbs a second year in a role, perhaps then they will begin to think about exercising. Of the adults who actually start walking, only a few will stay with it (Boone 2017).

This is where the ASEP Board-Certified Exercise Physiologist can help motivate individuals to stay with the exercise program, particularly from the point of view that exercise is medicine. Like most medicines, it should be taken with caution. Exercise physiologists are educated to help their clients and patients understand the physiologic responses to exercise, but they need the help of the medical community (Boone 2016a). This point is important, given that it provides meaning and purpose to prescribing exercise medicine and to the repetitious physical acts of walking around the block or lifting weights. The exercise physiologist can help keep the exercise response centered within one's own being, without which there is often the lack of desire to continue exercising. Because of this thinking, clients and patients need to be educated about the physiologic responses that are specific to exercise medicine (Boone 2017).

## References

*American Society of Exercise Physiologists*. (2019a). *Standards of Practice* [Online]. www.asep.org/index.php/organization/practice/

*American Society of Exercise Physiologists*. (2019b). *Home Page* [Online]. www.asep.org

Boone, T. (2013). *Introduction to Exercise Physiology*. Burlington, MA: Jones & Bartlett Publishing.

Boone, T. (2016a). Nothing Will Change Unless Physicians and Exercise Physiologists Start to Think Differently. *Journal of Exercise Medicine-Online*. 1(4);1–9.

Boone, T. (2016b). *ASEP's Exercise Medicine Text for Exercise Physiologists*. Sharjah, UAE: Bentham Science Publishers.

Boone, T. (2017). The Role of the Board-Certified Exercise Physiologist Is to Explain the Physiologic Responses of Exercise Medicine. *Journal of Exercise Medicine-online*. 2(1);1–6.

Boone, T. (2018). Diligence, Exercise Medicine, the Exercise Pill, and Career Success as an Exercise Physiologist: A Personal Perspective. *Journal of Exercise Medicine-online*. 3(2);15–26.

Booth, FW, Roberts, CK, Laye, MJ. (2012). Lack of Exercise is a Major Cause of Chronic Diseases. *Comparative Physiology*. 2(3);1143–1211.

# 14

# THE FUTURE OF FRAILTY

Individuals of all ages, especially 65 and over, must create the will to do something that will change their lives to help them be healthier. Instead of sitting all day and playing with the phone and other electronic stuff they have become enslaved to, they must develop the will to think beyond the moment. Yes, of course, no one is forcing anyone to stand up and begin an exercise program and, therefore, most adults don't move from the computer, the TV, or the couch, which is the problem. Most people are waiting for someone to push them because they are too lazy to get up and go for a 30-min walk and/or engage in some resistance training program. The sedentary lifestyle is not a healthy way to live. Statistically speaking, it results in premature diseases and death.

Individually and collectively, every person must become responsible for decreasing the incidence of his or her own disease and death. It is not logical to blame the boss or the fact that life is challenging. Yes, without question, work, friends, and anxiety can certainly distract a person from getting out of bed and going for a walk, but ultimately it is each person's responsibility to do the right thing for the right reason.

## Lifestyle: Drugs or Exercise Medicine

Without taking responsibility for an unhealthy lifestyle, adults cannot expect to live a healthy, long, or disease-free life. When properly prescribed by a healthcare professional (such as an ASEP Board-Certified Exercise Physiologist), regular exercise pushes the outer limits of life to enjoy more years of happiness and security in their relationship with family and friends. Exercise medicine is the personal means to achieving a healthier life, but more often than not adults of all ages fail to think about it or simply turn a deaf ear to the exercise medicine message.

It isn't front-page news that people have the freedom to watch TV or engage in exercise, or eat everything they can get their hands on or consume fewer calories, but with the freedom to do as one please comes responsibility. What would you do if you finally realized that you are sitting most of the hours of the day? Would you take responsibility for your sarcopenia? Think about it. It is obviously self-gratifying to say, "Yes, without a doubt I would get up from my

DOI: 10.4324/9781003119920-18

comfortable chair every 4 or 5 hours and go for a walk around the building that I work in or the homes in my neighborhood where I live. I want to be healthy." Well, when asked by a friend at work, "If that is the case, why is it that you are 60 lbs overweight? You know the extra weight isn't healthy." After some hesitation, John said,

> Obstacles keep getting in my way. Life isn't easy. My work is hard. It is complicated, but I need it to pay the bills. Yet, I am not sure from one day to the next whether I will have a job here next year.

---

**BOX 14.1 SETBACKS ARE PART OF LIFE. STAY THE COURSE.**

"Obstacles cannot crush me, every obstacle yields to stern resolve. He who is fixed to a star does not change his mind."

—Leonardo da Vinci

---

Many adults may think they are acting in their own best interest, but talking about exercising and actually exercising are two different things altogether. John knew that exercise is good for the mind and body, but nonetheless he continued to sit hour after hour watching TV at home in the evenings and weekends, eating relentlessly large amounts of food, and failing to deal with his stress at work. The problem of aging and physical inactivity goes beyond knowing what is right. It is a critical matter of doing what is right. Believe it, not because you are reading it, but because it is the truth (Boone, 2016).

The majority of Americans and people around the world have no idea how to develop the right attitude to put themselves in motion to conquer their problematic lifestyle. And yet, there are thousands of scientific papers that speak to the benefits of exercise medicine. They can be read by anyone, not just someone with a Ph.D. The content is clear in what it says, which is to get beyond the sedentary lifestyle and avoid chronic diseases and/or frailty. Exercise medicine is the means to putting people of all ages in charge of their lives. After all, adults of all ages, including the non-frail and elderly frail adults who engage in regular exercise, are less likely to live with a decline in their health, and those who are frail are more likely to live longer with less health issues.

## Attitude Makes the Difference

A person's attitude toward the exercise medicine prescription will make all the difference in the world. In fact, isn't it obvious that everything in life that is important depends on the person's attitude and willingness to take control of what he or she thinks and does? For example, if you should say, "I am going to be happy today," then, regardless of what happens throughout the day, there is an excellent chance you will handle the event or situation in a way that allows for you to be happy. We don't have to be unhappy or predisposed to chronic diseases more than normal. We can develop the attitude that we are responsible for being disciplined enough to believe in our inner voice. Call it faith or inspiration in positive thinking that gives a person the assurance of things hoped for, that is, the freedom from disease and/or negative thinking.

Attitude makes the difference, and no doubt you have heard this same message many times before. Why not expose yourself to a new way of thinking? Why not start today by saying, "I believe I can make a difference in my life by contacting a Board-Certified Exercise Physiologist who will develop an exercise medicine program specifically for me?" Why not say it again, "I believe I can and I will strengthen my cardiorespiratory system and my musculoskeletal system to avoid frailty and all of its health issues."

To press the point one more time, just recently a person was heard saying to one of his co-workers that he should start an exercise program to lose the 35 pounds he had gained during the past 2 years. His friend said, "I'm not interested. I don't want to exercise. I don't want to move from my computer. Exercise is boring, and I am not an athlete. Why do I have to lose weight anyway?" Then, out of the blue, the person got exasperated and said firmly,

> Well, I'll give you three reasons you have to start exercising. First, it is the right thing to do for your health, well-being, and family. Second, you are 60 yrs old and you are already looking frail. Third, you have high blood pressure.

The question is this: "Do you want to be bored or dead?" It is hard to overstate the importance of thinking differently, especially when it comes down to life or death.

## Exercise or Disease?

Yes, exercise medicine is regular exercise, but it is much more! It can be boring, difficult, and mentally a separation from moments of otherwise apparent comfort and/or relaxation with a person's computer or TV. But one significant statistic is that ~1 million people have a heart attack (i.e., myocardial infarction) every year in the United States. Those who have heart disease and related chronic diseases that promote the deterioration of the cardiovascular system are on the short course to flying without an engine, riding in a boat that is letting in water far from the shore, or walking across a busy street without looking both ways. Those who understand this point are often distressed by the individual or family member who looks the other way to the warning signs that exercise is imperative for sound health and well-being.

What else can a person say when speaking with a friend who isn't interested in understanding just how serious it is to turn a blind eye to his or her reality? How does a person build self-esteem in his friend, especially since it reflects on the individual's self-worth? The right answer to the question is very important.

Self-esteem is a reflection of a person's emotional state. For example, does he take pride in how he looks (e.g., the clothes he wears to work)? Yes, there are frail older adults who are still working. Does he respect himself and, if so, why isn't he acting in a responsible manner for himself and his family? Hanging tough in this world within a disease-driven reality by one's own self-imposed limitations isn't the answer to living a healthier lifestyle. Yes, there are times when it is necessary to break out of the "box" of a person's limitations to live a better life.

Everything about life and living from one day to the next with the worst of comments by friends, the lack of any desire to control one's caloric consumption throughout the day and night, and poor choices and attitudes that leave a person failing at work, at home, and elsewhere, older adults can find themselves on the short end of possibilities and opportunities that leave them feeling defeated. So, what is the point of believing a person can or should change the direction of his or her life? In short, why exercise? Larry was overheard saying,

> It makes little sense to me. Frankly, life is what it is. Some people are rich and some are poor. Some are healthy and strong while others are sick and frail. That is life. I don't think I can influence the outcome, so I live it to be as happy as I can. That means I consume as much food as I want to, drink alcohol regularly from the end of a day's work to when I go to sleep, and I do so while living constantly inside the world of my 75-inch television. It would be impossible for me to change, so why try? After all, I read that there are many research papers with conclusions that are made up lies and/or misconceptions of relationships between research variables.

Obviously, most people are hard to convince that exercise is the medicine of choice to prevent chronic diseases and frailty. They refuse to believe that exercise is medicine. It is their moment of intentional inattention. They refuse to take responsibility, regardless of the scientific papers and healthcare professionals that assert otherwise. Therefore, ultimately, each person has a choice. He or she can draw closer to the understanding that exercise is as vital, if not more so, than brushing one's teeth every morning. Or, the aging adult can keep his or her distance from a resistance training program and accept frailty with aging. Every person can choose either to be healthy and strong with an exercise medicine prescription or he or she can conclude that there isn't anything humanly possible to do and, therefore, accept the likelihood of getting old, weak, and miserable.

---

**BOX 14.2 THE PRACTICE OF EXERCISE MEDICINE BY EXERCISE PHYSIOLOGISTS.**

Healthy lifestyle requirements include stress management, regular exercise, and a sound diet. The practice of exercise physiology combines scientific thinking that underlies all three areas of concern. The risk of cardiovascular death is lower as physical activity levels are increased to prevent a health problem before it happens. Exercise physiology is similar to the practice of medicine, although certainly not the same. Exercise physiologists are not medical doctors, and medical doctors are not exercise physiologists. Even when medical doctors express an interest in the prescription of exercise, its application should exist with exercise physiologists, as is true for medication prescriptions with physicians. Rather than waiting for collaboration with the medical community, the exercise physiology profession should declare exercise as a powerful primary and secondary healthcare intervention that can and should be marketed by exercise physiologists.

**Disclosure:** Part of Chapter 14 was previously published in the article entitled The Will to Live in the *Journal of Exercise Medicine-online*. 2018;3(3):1–5.

---

## Final Thoughts

Board-Certified Exercise Physiologists recognize that they don't know everything about health and wellness. But frequently, they ask important questions about medicine, exercise, and professionalism. They have made a major effort to understand the role of a profession-specific organization and its influence on the size of their thinking, which is consistent with the ASEP perspective. The reason is because they think differently from the everyday exercise physiologists. There is evidence that supports their big-picture thinking, which is primarily witnessed by the time they took to study for and pass the "Certified Exercise Physiologist" exam. They are not satisfied with the thinking of a generic organization. Rather, they are more interested in enlarging their understanding and thinking about exercise physiology from the professional healthcare perspective that has provided them the education and the laboratory skills to help others become all they can be by living a life beyond wallowing in mediocrity?

As Jeremy Morris, the British epidemiologist wrote in 1982, "Exercise is today's best buy in public health" (Morris 1992). ASEP leaders are in position to take the leadership role in the recommendation and individualized prescriptive use of exercise medicine to prevent and treat frailty. Thus, when a patient is diagnosed with frailty, it is best that he or she is treated by a physician and an ASEP Board-Certified Exercise Physiologist who can help deal with the "how to" regarding the three exercise training programs. The exercise physiologist will help the elderly frail make the right decision to correct bad habits and misplaced thinking. They will help the adult turn his or her life around and take charge. Now is the time to get with the exercise medicine program. Remember, as Robert H. Schuller said, "It takes guts to leave the ruts."

## References

Boone, T. (2016). *ASEP's Exercise Medicine Text for Exercise Physiologists*. Sharjah, UAE: Bentham Science Publishers.

Morris, JN. (1992). Exercise versus Health Attack: History of a Hypothesis. In: Marmot, M, Elliot, P (Editors), *Coronary Heart Disease Epidemiology: From Aetiology to Public Health*. Oxford: Oxford Medical Publications.

# EPILOGUE

## Maximizing Health

A major responsibility of Board-Certified Exercise Physiologists is to help the elderly adults realize their full potential by avoiding frailty. This is a major healthcare responsibility because in the last 100 years, the populations in developed countries have experienced an unprecedented increase of 30 years in life expectancy. While the exercise physiologist's role in aging and frailty is not going to happen overnight, it must happen because a compression of morbidity and frailty could unleash a new life stage in which a healthy older population makes significant contributions to societal well-being and productivity (Fried 2018).

"Exercise medicine" is medicine prescribed by exercise physiologists. It is known to prevent and treat underlying frailty dysregulation of the physiologic systems that is considered a new medical syndrome (Morley et al. 2013). As a relatively new medical treatment, it is not a new concept and it does not have to be vigorous to have positive benefits (Xue et al. 2012). The medical dimension of exercise medicine improves sarcopenia and protein synthesis (Zampieri et al. 2015), improves glucose metabolism and inflammation, maintains mitochondrial function, prevents the release of reactive oxygen species, preserves slow-type fibers and muscle function, and improves oxidative muscle metabolism. Exercise medicine for the frailty syndrome breaks new ground by improving homeostasis and functionality (Fried 2018).

The challenges of maximizing health of aging adults are multifaceted. To begin with, it should go without saying that the medical community must aim to include frailty assessment tools as inclusion criteria (Theou et al. 2011) to understand the elderly frail adult's health issues. The physician must evaluate whether aging adults are consuming sufficient proteins, calories, and essential nutrients for the prevention and treatment of frailty. Then, with referral to an exercise physiologist, the exercise medicine component can be implemented as a medicine to help with frailty. The main purpose of the multi-pronged approach is to prevent or delay the progression of frailty and the associated functional decline with aging. This means that in addition to aging adults being treated by a physician, geriatric nurse specialist, nutritionist, and physical therapist among others, they should also be supervised by an exercise physiologist to help prevent or slow the progression of frailty and increase independent living (Boone & Foley 1997).

Other challenges increase numerous negative effects, such as the functional decline that makes it difficult to withstand or rebound from falls, disabilities, and chronic illnesses, all resulting

DOI: 10.4324/9781003119920-19

in readmission to hospitals. The healthcare challenges not only include decisions about the right medical treatment but also how to access and pay for daily care, medications, nutritional concerns, travel to and from healthcare appointments and housing in nursing facilities, retirement housing, adult day care, and exercise medicine programs.

In 2000, the U.S. government spent $585 billion on health care. About 66% of that amount was spent on older adults (Young 2003). It is hard to imagine where they get the money. Newton-Small (2019) had this to say,

> Caring for America's elders is the single most expensive domestic priority on the horizon, breaking the projected budgets of both Medicare and Medicaid, all 50 states and most of the middle class, and the truth is, no one is truly prepared for what is to come (Box 1).

---

**BOX EPILOGUE 1.1  HEALTH CARE FOR FRAIL OLDER ADULTS.**

Frail older adults "have a higher frequency of primary care visits, consume 50% of all hospital care, and use over 80% of home care services, and occupy 90% of all nursing home beds in the United States."

—Mezey, M, Fulmer, T. (1998). Quality Care for the Frail Elderly. *Nursing Outlook.* 46(6);291–292.

---

While concerns abound regarding appropriate prevention and treatment of the elderly frail adult, it is expected that there will be an increase in delivery of home and community-based services as alternatives to nursing homes and more costly levels of care. One solution that will gain more attention from individuals and family members who reach out to their physician to access help from an exercise physiologist to bring hopeful relief to the frail older adult. The exercise medicine delivery of care will become recognized as a credible alternative to nursing home care and reliance on traditional hospital care, medications, and hospital-based technologies.

There will still be a professional relationship between the two care systems. But the exercise physiology system will provide the medical exercise intervention and assessments to enhance quality of life and functional abilities of older adults. Portable laboratory equipment will be used to explain relevant information, to provide treatment care, to educate the frail adults, and to promote optimal care in their homes or that of the family caregivers. The expected outcome is the potential to promote independence, dignity, and autonomy among frail elders (Box 2).

---

**BOX EPILOGUE 1.2  THE EXERCISE PHYSIOLOGISTS' ROLE IN PROMOTING HEALTHY AGING.**

Improving outcomes for frail older adults start with recognizing exercise physiologists as part of the primary care team to improve health, delay disability, and increase well-being. The future of ASEP Board-Certified Exercise Physiologists is linked to the expectation that exercise medicine and its role in promoting a healthier older population. This

> expectation, led by the ASEP's Exercise Physiologists' Standards of Professional Practice, is a shared commitment with family caregivers and healthcare professionals to promote optimal clinical outcomes, functional ability, and quality of life in the elderly frail adults.

The increase in delivery of home and community-based services for the elderly frail adults will help with their complex health issues that make it difficult for them to travel to a clinic for care. Seeing clients and/or patients in the comfort and privacy of their own home will also allow for safety assessments of the home environment in addition to an accurate assessment of medications and functional assessment. The home setting will also allow for spending more time with the elderly adult, allowing for a more open discussion around the patient's most pressing questions and concerns as well as exploring his or her hopes, fears, and overall goals of care.

As a treatment area, the home visit is unique in that it provides the opportunity for the exercise physiologist to see, experience, and discuss the implementation of the exercise medicine prescription. Also, there is the close-up opportunity to identify the challenges that may exist when walking in the community, what to anticipate, how to plan ahead, and how to stay in contact with exercise physiologist regarding any concerns about the prescription. Home visits will provide increased opportunity to identify adults who are just beginning to demonstrate qualities of becoming frail. Hence, it is very important that the client or patient's physician, in particular, assumes a major responsibility in how they relate to and treat exercise physiologists as healthcare professionals.

## References

Boone, T, Foley, M. (1997). Aging and Performance. In: *Encyclopedia of Sports Science* (Volume 2), New York, NY: Simon & Schuster Macmillan.

Fried, LP. (2018). Interventions for Human Frailty: Physical Activity as a Model. *Cold Spring Harbor Perspective Medicine.* 6(6);1–14.

Mezey, M, Fulmer, T. (1998). Quality Care for the Frail Elderly. *Nursing Outlook.* 46(6);291–292.

Morley, JE, Vellas, B, Abellan van Kan G, et al. (2013). Frailty Consensus: A Call to Action. *Journal of American Medical Directors Association.* 14;392–397.

Newton-Small, J. (2019). A Growing American Crisis: Who Will Care for the Baby Boomers? *Time* [Online]. https://time.com/5529152/elderly-caregiving-baby-boomers-unpaid-caregivers-crisis/

Theou, O, Stathokostas, L, Roland, KP, et al. (2011). The Effectiveness of Exercise Interventions for the Management of Frailty: A Systematic Review. *Journal of Aging Research.* Article ID 569194, 19 pages.

Xue, QL, Bandeen-Roche, K, Mielenz, TJ, et al. (2012). Patterns of 12-Year Change in Physical Activity Levels in Community-Dwelling Older Women: Can Modest Levels of Physical Activity Help Older Women Live Longer? *American Journal of Epidemiology.* 176;534–543.

Young, HM. (2003). Challenges and Solutions for Care of Frail Older Adults. *The Online Journal of Issues in Nursing.* 2;1–13.

Zampieri, S, Pietrangelo, L, Loefler, S, et al. (2015). Lifelong Physical Exercise Delays Age-Associated Skeletal Muscle Decline. *Journal of Gerontology: A Biological Science and Medical Sciences.* 70;163–173.

# INDEX

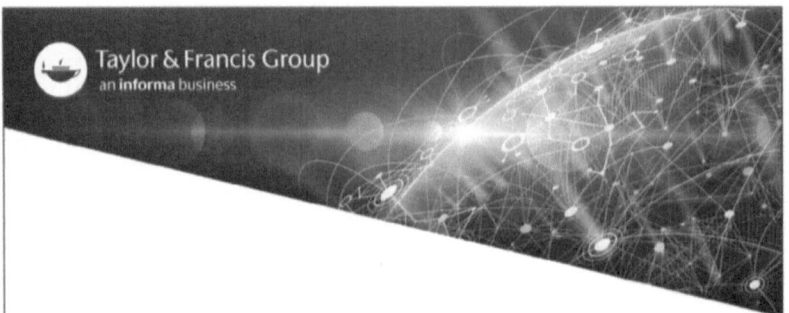
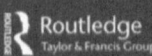
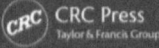